I Have MS.
What's Your Super Power?

A Common Sense Guide to Living With MS

Lisa A. McCombs

Headline Books, Inc.
Terra Alta, WV

I Have MS. What's Your Super Power?

by Lisa A. McCombs

©2016 Lisa A. McCombs

Headline Books, Inc.
P. O. Box 52
Terra Alta, WV 26764
www.headlinebooks.com
Tel: 800-570-5951
Email: mybook@headlinebooks.com

LisaAnnetteMcCombs@yahoo.com

Lisa A. McCombs
358 McCue Avenue
Monongah, WV 26554

Cover illustration by Ashley Teets
www.AshleyTeetsIllustration.com

ISBN 9781882658442

Library of Congress Control Number: 2015951677

PRINTED IN THE UNITED STATES OF AMERICA

Dedicated to my little sister, a fellow MSer, who fought the good fight. Jamie, we are not finished yet. Thank you for cheering us on from Heaven.

Prologue

I remember watching episodes of Batman on my family's small black and white television. I loved the animated Pow! Bang! Zap! that illustrated the emotion of action. The Bat Cave became my fantasy home and who didn't want the blind loyalty of a protégé like Robin.

Later, I discovered Superman, and Clark Kent fast became my super hero of choice. A relative orphan sent to earth in order to live a human life with super human powers. As long as Superman steered clear of his nemesis kryptonite, he could do anything.

In dealing with Multiple Sclerosis, we need to be aware of our personal kryptonite and work hard to keep it at bay. I believe that Common Sense can be just about the most powerful weapon in our super power arsenal. So, I have chosen Common Sense to be my partner in fighting the ill effects of MS. It is not a cure. It does not eliminate physical pain nor does it work miracles. But if we employ a daily dose of Common Sense, we can turn this MonSter into a super power worth reckoning with.

I hope that in sharing my thoughts on multiple sclerosis, that you, my readers and fellow warriors, will discover your personal kryptonite(s) and know how to battle the MonSter.

We are super heroes. We have MS.

That is our super power.

MS is basically an attack on the immune system. With that in mind, identifying our individual kryptonite is a matter of listening to our body.

So, warriors, arm yourself with the knowledge and face your kryptonite head-on.

My Name is Multiple Sclerosis

by Leslie Hillburn, Founder of the Face Book page, We're Not Drunk, We Have MS!

Hi, my name is MS and I'm an invisible chronic illness. I am now velcroed to you for life. Others around you can't see me or hear me, but YOUR body feels me. I can attack you anywhere and anyhow I please. I can cause severe pain, or, if I'm in a good mood, I can just cause you to ache all over.

Remember when you and Energy ran around together and had fun? I took Energy from you and gave you Exhaustion. Try to have fun now! I also took Good Sleep from you and in its place gave you Brain Fog. I can make you tremble internally, or make you feel cold or hot when everyone else feels normal. Oh yeah, I can make you feel anxious or depressed, too. If you have something planned or are looking forward to a great day, I can take that away, too. You didn't ask for me. I chose you for various reasons: that virus you had that you never recovered from, or that car accident, or maybe it was the years of abuse and trauma. Well, anyway, I'm here to stay!

I hear you're going to see a doctor who can get rid of me. I'm rolling on the floor laughing! Just try. You will have to go to many, many doctors until you find one who can help you effectively. You will be put on pain pills, sleeping pills, energy pills; told you are suffering from anxiety or depression, given a TENS unit, get massaged, told if you just sleep and exercise properly I will go away; told to think positively, poked, prodded, and MOST OF ALL, not taken as seriously as you feel when you cry to the doctor how debilitating life is every day.

Your family, friends, and coworkers will all listen to you until they just get tired of hearing about how I make you feel and that I'm a debilitating disease. Some of them will say things like "Oh, you are just having a bad day" or "Well, I can't do the things I used to do 20

YEARS ago," not hearing that you said 20 DAYS ago. Some will just start talking behind your back, while you slowly feel you are losing your dignity trying to make them understand, especially when you are in the middle of a conversation with a "Normal" person and can't remember what you were going to say next!

In closing, (I was hoping that I kept this part a secret, but I guess that you already found out!)....the ONLY place you will get any support and understanding in dealing with me is with Other People With MS.

Chapter One

The Long Walk Home

Finally! The beginning of summer vacation. The day that every public school student and their teachers have looked forward to since mid-August. For me, this summer held an even more special ingredient. In two weeks, my newborn would celebrate six months on this earth and we had the entire summer to play, learn, and laugh, starting with this morning's mile-long walk to the public library. He would enjoy the stroller ride and I could begin to document his academic beginnings.

I stocked the stroller with bagged apple slices, yummy kiddie cookies and bottled water, my library card, sunscreen and a spare diaper. My walking routine had been traded in for feeding schedules and mommy duties lately, so I looked forward to this hike for more than one reason. My legs were getting lazy and my Reeboks were looking too clean.

I spread a thin layer of extra strength sun block on baby's face, secured his new Old Navy ball cap, and lowered the stroller visor to ensure that harmful rays were filtered. My own sun hat was in place and sunglasses secured.

We set out with the sun to our backs and I made certain to comment on the sights of downtown Fairmont as we crossed traffic and entered the more historic portion of our small city. The morning was clear and traffic was light, so our journey was the perfect way to begin what promised to be the perfect summer sojourn from academia.

An hour later, with a stroller full of colorful children's books for baby and two crime novels for me, I carefully tucked my now-sleeping son back into his chariot and began the return walk home. The sun was a little higher and its rays noticeably warmer, but it felt good. I was on top of the world.

Life couldn't get much better than this, I remember thinking and wished for the umpteenth time I knew how to whistle. This just seemed like the perfect moment to let out a light-hearted whistle. I had the perfect child. This was a perfect morning, very near a perfect library, the perfect distance away for the perfect morning stroll.

And then, as with all perfect plans, the bottom fell out and all hell broke loose. Four city blocks from home, my vision suddenly blurred and my right arm began to tingle in a strange, limb-falling-asleep manner. For some reason I could no longer fully lift my right foot and my mouth felt like it was actually pulled down in what I imagined was a comic book grimace.

The sun was really beating down on us by then and there were no shady places to rest for a moment and try to collect myself. This was really, really weird. If it was just me, I could crawl home. I would fit right in with the street folks who vacated the empty shop-door wells on the upper end of town. But it wasn't just me. I looked down at my little miracle and attempted to adjust the stroller visor, but my arms were becoming strangely useless and I decided to conserve my strength for crossing the highway

I'll have a drink. That's the ticket. I remember focusing on that water bottle with such an intensity that I had hoped to will it to rise up to me and rinse me in its refreshing contents. But it didn't. Remember? My perfect morning, my perfect plan was no longer perfect, so any magical, lifesaving actions were safely resting in the stacks back in the fantasy section of the library.

I remember staring out at the four lane (thankfully not polluted with traffic, yet) and praying to God I could safely push my son's stroller to the other side. My legs were so weak and my right foot had to be practically dragged.

At least the wheels on the stroller would help pull me in the right direction.

I stepped off that curb and plunged my son and myself into the middle of the highway, steeling myself to ignore the angry car horns that surprisingly did not sound. Or maybe there were none. I really do not know. This portion of my return walk home has gone to the selective portion of my brain, for which I am grateful. I really do not want to know how we crossed that highway. It's more important that we did.

To this day I do not know exactly how I managed to cross that street to complete my journey over the uneven sidewalk to my own front porch. One concrete step up to the front walk and two porch steps to reach the front door elude me. I do remember sitting on the front step beside my sleeping baby, wondering how on earth I was going to move that stroller to the front door. I was terrified at the prospect of lifting my child in my numb arms and actually carrying him the distance to the door. By now I couldn't feel the fingers on my left hand and my right arm hung uselessly at my side.

Someone was watching over me that day. Of that there is no question. I think I might have dozed there in the shade of my front yard pine tree because the next memory I have is that of my son making small, conversational noises from his stroller seat. Without even thinking I reached for him and rose from my perch to carry him inside, away from the heat.

It was as if my horrible walk home had never happened. I had to stretch my imagination to recall the frightening events of the afternoon, but I would not be convinced otherwise. And, of course, as paranormal fate would have it, the lack-of-sensations returned as soon as I changed and fed my son.

It wasn't as bad, but it was there, what ever it was. I knew that medical attention was absolutely essential. The only physician I knew to contact was my OBGYN, who blessedly granted me an emergency visit. His advice—Go to the ER, straight to the ER, do not pass GO, do not collect $200. This was no post-natal event, but I could tell he had his suspicions.

I got some flack from my then spouse, but I had a new reason to take care of myself. I hadn't planned to be a mother at the age of 40. Nor had I any plans to contract some lethal disease.

Upon registration into the hospital, I was poked, prodded, x-rayed, cat-scanned, and MRI'd. Extensive tests ruled out a stroke and there was no conclusive evidence of any other sensible condition. The entire time I spent in the hospital my biggest concern was the welfare of my child. My mother was out of town and I didn't want to worry my father. Being of an advanced age for a young mother, I didn't have any friends around who were free to help me out.

I finally called a relatively close girl friend whose work allowed her a little more freedom than most people and she agreed to hook up with my husband and lend a hand. (They ended up married a few short years later.) Until recently, I thought my son was in her care exclusively until my brother and sister-in-law informed me their baby nephew had spent quality time in their hands. To this day I am still filling in the gaps.

Eleven days later I returned home to continue my summer vacation.

I relearned how to walk, feed myself, and enunciate words. I couldn't hold my child without fear of dropping him. On July 1, 2001, I had a spinal tap and was officially diagnosed with relapsing-remitting multiple sclerosis. I was prescribed Beta Seron. I learned how to self-inject and I dealt with it. My son's favorite movie became my VHS instructional video on how to inject Beta Seron. To this day we laugh about it. I fear I will be forced to convert that old VHS to a DVD for his eighteenth birthday! If he chooses a career in medicine, I can blame it on that video.

My real MS adventure began that summer. My first lesson was to find out what MS was and how long I had to live. Morbid? Yes. Unrealistic? No.

Well, that was nearly fifteen years ago and I am still kicking, but the true definition of MS remains a mystery to me and will probably remain so until my final breath.

Chapter Two

Water Works

Incontinence.

A friend of mine used this word once in describing strange physical symptoms she was experiencing. Due to her habitual hypochondriac tendencies, as well as the fact the word was alien to my vocabulary, I really didn't think much of it at the time. I just nodded in requisite acknowledgment and let her continue to vent.

I have had to learn to deal with many humiliations prior to being diagnosed with MS, but this is the most alarming.

When the word popped up again during D-Day (Diagnosis Day), my mind raced to recall the first time I had ever heard it. I immediately cringed in sympathy for anyone who experienced such a degrading, animalistic situation.

And, then, I realized that I HAD experienced incontinence, but I had associated it with a probable urinary tract infection for which I was prone. Wow, two red flags all at once, but I didn't know how closely these situations were related or what they had in common.

Incontinence is one of the biggest problems I have with my disease. It is not uncommon for me to not quite make it to the toilet on time or even know that I need to go in time to even think about searching for said toilet.

In the beginning, and even now, I am not comfortable in strange settings if I haven't located the ladies' room and have developed an acceptable escape route just in case. There are particular places I refuse to visit because I know, without a doubt, that disaster lurks. When my favorite grocery store got a face lift and removed the public restrooms, I no longer shopped there. I only shop at stores that offer close proximity to a public restroom and I only try on clothes after several visits to the lady's room.

Pre-diagnosis I can remember sitting in traffic and feeling my bladder totally empty onto the plush black upholstery of my snazzy l'il sports car.

It was a warm day. I had driven several miles aware of a need to relieve myself but confident I could and would make it to the next fast food restroom, located right up the road. That's when the traffic lights failed me and progress toward those Golden Arches stopped. Thank goodness I was alone, with no witnesses. (That has not always been the case.)

I hated to soil my car seat but at least this hadn't happened in someone else's vehicle! (Eww...) I could clean this up with no one the wiser, even if the chore took precedence over my evening plans of driving to a friend's house. (Double eww...I didn't relish the idea of plopping myself back down in my own pee.) And right now I needed to get home and clean myself up. Sitting in my own puddle was not a pleasant sensation.

Why had this happened? What was wrong with my body that I couldn't "hold my water"?

Afterward, I remember laughing at myself as if I had committed a secret blunder to lock away in my private memory vault.

But then it happened again...and again...and again...

Once at a deli...once in the hallway at school...no, twice...no, three times at school...once on my back porch as I fumbled for the house key...again in my kitchen after miscalculating the number of steps it would take to reach the bathroom...once in line at Walmart...a couple of times in bed...when I stood up at my desk...on the edge of a ski boat (but that was okay since I was already wet and in the river)...

You get the picture.

What horrid fuel for an already accelerated anxiety level. I never knew when it would happen and I began avoiding consumption of liquids to the point of near hydration. The muscles that controlled that physical act of waiting no longer obeyed my command. I envisioned a bladder bag attached to my side or packages of adult diapers stacked in my linen closet.

My gynecologist suggested practicing Kegle exercises daily. My mother told me to wear Depends (That figures!). My urologist prescribed an assortment of medicines and with each failed prescription changed it to another. My neurologist just told me I would have to live with it. This was all after D-Day, so you can only imagine the assistance I received without a definitive medical condition.

I admit that I really didn't do much (any) research on my situation after diagnosis. It was what it was.

Boy, oh, boy, have I learned to lean on myself since then. If I want to know, I need to Google it! Since my diagnosis, my life has taken a new direction. I still teach full-time; I am a mother and a wife; I enjoy my hobbies of reading, writing, and crocheting; I attend church and play in the bell choir; but I do not go out of my way to look for additional responsibilities. I enjoy my home, my books, and my teaching. And I head for the lavatory at the first sensation, no matter how small.

I'm sure there is a pill out there with my name on it that would alleviate this problem, but I am also certain that pill would only lead to another problem that requires prescription treatment, so I will pass and once again take matters into my own hands. I do that a lot.

In fact, I have found that living with multiple sclerosis requires a lot of self-experimentation. The MonSter treats its members differently. What works for one MSer may not be the answer for another. I wish I had kept a journal to detail my journey from day one, but hindsight doesn't do me any good right now. So, to throw around yet another overly used cliché, there is no time like the present.

Things I have learned about living with MS:

*Stay out of the heat.

*Always know the fastest and most direct path to a bathroom.

*Have a walking device (my poison is a cane) close, even when you are feeling your strongest.

*Always know the fastest and most direct path to a bathroom.

*Stay hydrated.

*Always know the fastest and most direct path to a bathroom.

*Exercise daily.

*Engage in a hobby, or two, or three.

*Do not apologize for your disability. Remember: it only disables you if you allow it.

*Find an outreach group, either on line or face-to-face.

*Wear comfortable shoes.

*Always know the fastest and most direct path to a bathroom.

Chapter Three

Coffee, tea, or glatiramer acetate?

I hate drugs. I hate them, I hate them, I do. The older I get, the more my disdain grows, but unfortunately, the more chemicals I am forced to feed into my body.

Upon diagnosis, my neuro selected Beta Seron from the three newest MS treatments on the market. Beta Seron was the least invasive at the time. I injected every other day according to a rotating skin location schedule. The needle is very small and relatively painless. In the beginning I injected manually. The auto injector made things a whole lot easier.

I used Beta Seron for eleven years before just deciding to stop. That winter a major snow storm turned into a governor-issued state-of-emergency that blocked road travel of any kind. It lasted for nearly a week.

School children celebrated with the cancellation of schools. Area businesses suffered from lack of economy. And I could not get to the pharmacy to pick up my meds.

I'm sure other arrangements might have been made if I had treated this as a medical emergency, but I didn't. End of story.

I was drug free (except for an assortment of pain killers and infection fighting steroids) for four years. I had no interest in experimenting with any more MS treatments. Life was good as long as I remembered to exercise a bit, get my rest, drink plenty of water and steer clear of stressful situations. By the time my neuro convinced me I owed it to my family to be proactive with my condition, I felt strong enough to do just that.

On December 24, 2014, I took my first dose of Tecfidera. The idea of an oral MS treatment was intriguing. No more injections, no more ugly skin irritations and injection schedules, no more needles…brilliant! A medical treatment so free and easy made Tecfidera the perfect choice in warding off further/frequent flare ups. This proved to me that research was finally progressing and an end to this horrible disease was near. An oral med! Go figure!

My husband and I had discussed this and he was in full support. Thank goodness. The darling man had no idea what he signed up for! Neither did I.

As forewarned, the side-effects of Tec were a tad (ha!) different than the flu-like symptoms promised with the early days of Beta Seron. I had never suffered any side-effects with Beta Seron, so I felt immune. And for the first nine days of taking Tecfidera, it looked as if my good fortune was a lasting thing.

The following is my day-to-day journal of life with Tecfiera, until the proverbial sh*! hit the fan.

Tecfidera - Day 2

Merry Christmas to all!

The flushing began this afternoon hours after swallowing my third dose of Tecfidera. It was awful. My skin (full body) turned a nice Christmas red and I felt like a swarm of fire ants had taken over as a new skin covering. I was hot to the touch and the chills set in for nearly an hour. It is difficult to separate the sensation from that of what my son is feeling with his holiday bout of the flu. Once the heat diminished and the chills abated, I felt certain it wasn't the flu (not yet, at least) and directed my panic to the internet to question other Tec users about my symptoms. It seems this is nothing unusual and I was gifted with several suggestions. I plan to take a baby aspirin twenty minutes prior to my next dose and was told to drink lots of water.

We'll see...

Other than my crazy pal MS and my son's flu, this has been a nice family day.

I have found that focusing on a passion, in this case journaling, is an important part of life and an even more essential part of living with an incurable disease. Y'see, when referred to that way, "incurable disease," it sounds rather important, doesn't it? And important situations surround important people, whether they are pissing themselves in Walmart or sitting on the royal throne at home. That is something to remember and focus upon while wrestling with your new companion. You are an important person with an important disease. You do important things.

Tecfidera - Day 4

Well, I am still breathing and am experiencing no weird symptoms other than the horrible flushing that seems to have abated—possibly due to the baby aspirin—possibly due to multiple doses and my body adapting to this new intrusion of chemicals. Such is the way with MS. Everything is an hypothesis (one of my students favorite vocabulary words as they find it comes in handy at times of class argument).

So, to clear up the mud a bit, "Tecfidera [dimethyl fumarate] is a prescription medicine used to treat people with relapsing forms of multiple sclerosis." Got that? Tells you everything needed, right?

Tecfidera is a pill form of MS treatment that is far less painful than the alternating-daily needle of Beta Seron that I once enjoyed. Just because it is less painful to consume makes it no less scary, though. I mean, putting any alien chemical in one's body is not and has never been on my bucket list of life experiences. I will admit that I like beer and thoroughly enjoy a glass or two of sweet wine, but that is actually as far as my chemical pleasures go. I am not a pill person and I avoid over the counter cold and sinus remedies if I can battle those situations with vitamin C, lots of liquids, and bed rest. So, this whole Tecfidera thing is not my normal MO.

Tecfidera, as with any MS medication, will not cure MS nor will it "make me better." What Tecfidera and all the other MS drugs do is (supposedly and hopefully) reduce the number of relapses (exasperations). According to my handy dandy Tecfidera user's guide "27%

of people taking Tecfidera experienced a relapse compared with 46% of people taking placebo, making them 49% less likely to experience a relapse.

This means that less than 3 out of 10 people taking Tecfidera experienced a relapse. I guess I am crazy, but I am less concerned about relapses than I am about what this drug is doing to my brain. Of course my user guide doesn't mention the rare, but possible, side effect of brain infection associated with this drug. Supposedly as long as my neuro keeps an eye on my white blood cell count things will be okay. My guide booklet tells me I can report any side effects to FDA at 1-800-FDA-1088 or for more information I can log on to dailymed.nlm.nig.gov. Reassuring, I know.

I apologize if my take on Tec is far too cynical for you, my reader. It's just a way of venting, I suppose. MS just sucks and, "that is all I'm going to say about that," (Forrest Gump), at least for now.

I did get a cute little pill box from Biogen, the pharmaceutical company that produces MS drugs. So, along with my growing collection of designer canes, I now have an attractive reminder to take my pills twice a day.

If you want to know more about Tecfidera, go to www.tecfidera.com and to learn more about multiple sclerosis, visit nationalMSociety.org.

Tecfidera - Day 5

I was a little worried this morning when I realized I had slept until nearly 9:30. My drug routine scheduled me to take my Tec at 8:00, but I swallowed a baby aspirin and prepared breakfast for my son and husband to give the aspirin a head start. After a bowl of Rice Chex and a cup of coffee I took dose 9 and I have suffered no side effects today. It's been a busy day and I am happy with my little accomplishments. I thoroughly cleaned my laundry room and shampooed the rug where the litter box is located. My cat's "space" is clean again. I hope she appreciates it.

When I was younger I used to take on cleaning projects with a vengeance, scrubbing, dusting, vacuuming, shining, tossing old stuff...I have discovered with a few years on me and the inconvenience of

MS that I am much more productive taking my tasks in small measure with little rests in between. So, after the basement cleaning, I picked up a borrowed library book and allowed Joy Fielding to suck me into one of her superbly written mysteries. I am actually surprised that I put it down long enough to warm up some leftovers for a light lunch.

My second planned project for the day was to tidy my desk area in preparation of the arrival of my new desk top computer. It should be here tomorrow and I am very excited to welcome this Christmas present to myself. I got a great deal on a refurbished Dell and have BIG writing plans for it.

After being on winter break since December 23, I realize that my tentative plan to retire at the end of the school year is actually a good idea. I love being home to pursue my writing passion.

I have an affection for routine, but last night I actually stayed up reading until 1:00 a.m. That's not like me and I do not plan to make it a habit, but I have to admit that I kinda like breaking the early-to-bed-early-to-rise rule to which school teachers adhere. No matter how adequately we mature in life, there is still a bit of that rebellious child lurking, isn't there?

Tecfidera - Days 6 and 7

Okay, it is happening, just as I anticipated, my blogging activity is just as lame as it was before I committed to chronicling (That's an awkward word, if it is even a word at all.) my Tecfidera journey. WVU, my favorite college team and one of my Alma Maters, played in the Liberty Bowl yesterday and demanded my attention. With husband and his good friend (and WVU buddy), we huddled around the big screen downstairs to "tailgate" with our Mountaineers. It was a heart breaking couple of hours, full of ups and downs, nacho chips, cold beer (Yep, I was a bad girl, but did my best to keep things under control.), and comradery (I have spell checked over and over again and I cannot find the correct spelling of this word, but I know it is a word!)

Anyway, here I am again after taking dose thirteen and on the last day of 120mg installments of this new and mysterious MS treatment. I am very nervous about "upping" the dose tomorrow to 240mg twice a day. I want to have faith in this pill so badly, but after living with no meds for three years and still functioning, I am just not extremely excited about filling my body with chemicals. I've read and shared the data, but it's rather ludicrous to throw all of your faith into studies comparing chemical and placebo use. Of course, there is probably no other way to conduct these studies. I just find it unnerving to compare written words to the actual human reactions.

Yep, I'm rambling, but I am no longer flushing. Will that happen again when I double the dose tomorrow? If MS is nothing else, it is extremely unpredictable, making it terribly exciting. Right?

When my family zip-lined during our vacation a few years ago I was elated to participate in such an extreme sport. That was exciting and so not like me. Can I compare my zip lining experience to living with MS? Because I would love to say that MS is not like me either, but MS is me. MS has made me re-evaluate my life.

My mother is constantly talking about "one of these days" and I suddenly realized that every day is actually "one of these days." I have to stop putting off what I can accomplish today. So, I zip-line and would actually like to do it again. This time through a National Forest. There are several things I would like to do. Oh, this is the eve of New Year's Eve, so I suppose it is a good time to talk about those things I would like to do. Because this is so spur of the moment, my resolution list may require future editing, but here goes:

* Find an agent for my nonfiction guide to living with MS. (Spoiler alert: The tentative working title is Bruised, but Not Broken)

* Retire from teaching (still up in the air about that one)

*Remodel the bathroom and put new carpet in my bedroom (So, very, very materialistic)

Enough...bored already!

I'm burning daylight hours with this nonsense anyway. I have a WVU basketball game to attend and a little time to spend with my gal pals after while. I promise to be a good girl today and to enjoy every single second.

See you tomorrow.

Tecfidera - Days 8 and 9

Happy New Year!

This is my second day on full dose 240mg twice a day. I was really nervous about doubling my dosage, but I actually made a very smooth transition yesterday and felt absolutely no side effects or weirdness. So, I guess I am officially a Teccie (Teckie? Techie?). I had really hoped to write this installment on my new desk top computer, but as my husband and I were hooking everything up, I realized why I gave up my last desk top. For some reason our desk tops require a USB adapter in order to access the internet and I gave mine to my son when he received his birthday present this year. So, I suppose I need to make a visit to our local Radio Shack in order to use my new possession. The biggest reason I purchased was the deal I got. Just hope it doesn't back fire as so many deals are prone to do. I will still need to find a laptop after the school year is over, but if I am going to devote hours to writing, I need to move my computer time from the couch with my laptop to another room with my desk top. Eliminating all distractions is one of my new year's resolutions.

(Whoa! News to me. I didn't realize that I had made resolutions until those words appeared on the screen. Isn't it interesting what happens when the fingers take over and there are no distractions?)

Well, today is the first day of 2015. When I was my son's age, I never would have imagined being here in the year 2015. Wow! When I was his age, the year was 1973. Disco wasn't even hot yet! And now I am entertaining retirement. The years, they certainly do race along. In that case, here is another resolution: I refuse to waste a second of this life. Every day has a gift and I plan to open every one that I have left with appreciation and great joy. When I think of it this way, I know I am ready for the next chapter in my life. And I embrace this new opportunity with excitement.

Want to know more about Tecfidera? Well, the flushing seems to have dissipated, for which I am extremely grateful and after reading more about it all, I realize I have also experienced a little nausea and diarrhea, but it has been so minute I will not dwell on that. My guide book says "stomach problems tend to happen earlier in treatment and usually decrease over time." That's encouraging. And it's good to know that there is an Active Nurse available at 1-800-456-2255.

We have a saying around my house, especially when a seemingly easy project fails. "When in doubt, read the directions." In this case, I should have read and re-read the side-effect warnings. On day ten, I was hugging the porcelain throne. Several hours after that, I was elevated to queen of that throne with the waste paper basket as my scepter. It appeared that my new role in life was that of Human Disposal.

After three days reign over the bathroom, I found the strength to drag myself up from the lovely ceramic tile floor of which I know now every detail. I love that floor. It was a high priority selling point when I bought my house, but too much of anything is not a good idea.

Being a Face Book junky, I knew there were several social media groups on line that dedicated themselves in assisting those of us with MS. These are excellent places to vent, ask questions, and share. (Hi, guys. You Are The Boss!) Every super hero needs back up, and I knew I could find it there.

Folks with MS love to tell their story and are always at the ready with first-hand advice and suggestions. In response to my Tecfidera experience, I was offered a plethora (I love that word) of responses, the main theory of which was to "hang in there." Many of the suggestions were uplifting. Some of them just not feasible.

I realize I must take care of myself in order to care for those I love, but Tecfidera just wasn't worth the sacrifices I faced. I could not take weeks from work in order to adjust to this new drug. My reaction to this drug was far too disturbing to continue. Within a month I had lost nearly fifteen pounds (not the best diet to entertain) and my energy level was sub-zero. Prior to Tecfidera, I exercised daily (not high impact aerobics, but I could at least move). Quality of life was deteriorating and I had no time in my life for that.

Common Sense won and I decided that Tecfidera was NOT for me.

In my research, I have found eighty-nine medical/prescribed treatments to battle the MonSter. Eighty-nine! That number just blows my mind. Of course, the majority of those are still in the experimental stage, just as most drugs on the market. There is no cure for death. The undeniable truth is that death even visits Super Heroes. I am not totally convinced that just because we have MS, it is necessary to be on a drug, but medical science is very convincing in providing MR images of brain and spine lesion activity to support pharmaceutical participation in the disease.

Sometimes even Super Heroes must choose a poison, so my most recent venture in MS-altering treatment is Copaxone. I'll give it a shot (pun intended) until my next MRI. Jamie, I'm doing this for you,

I hope it works.

There are so many options out there. It is disturbing, yet very exciting to know researchers are on task. Even in the mid-1950s, persons with multiple sclerosis (as yet unlabeled) were often institutionalized or left to deal with life on their own. At least medical science has recognized the MonSter as a legitimate condition and is working on a possible cure.

It is absolutely necessary to stay on top of your disease. Research, read, talk to others with MS. Be proactive. Don your super hero cape and fly!

A book I have found helpful is *Multiple Sclerosis for DUMMIES*. (Seriously, there is a for-DUMMIES book out there for everything!) Especially if you are newly diagnosed, it is a wonderful guide book.

Chapter Four

You're Just Not That Interesting Anymore

Okay, the sad but honest news is that having MS is a novelty that gets less interesting the longer it attempts to hang out with the crowd. The initial diagnosis receives rave reviews of "OMG! What can I do? If you ever need anything, I'm only a phone call away, or, Call me when you're feeling down. We'll talk."

That lasts for a few weeks, maybe months, and possibly the "'til death us part" participants may hang on for a few years. And then, reality sets in as MS begins to rob its victim of more and more abilities in exchange for more mundane hobbies and interests.

I was the party girl, always game for a cold drink and some quality socializing. And then, bang! My medication took precedence over beer and my life's purpose became focused on my health, my son, and my survival.

My routine centered on my injections and the possible side effects of each and every dose. I had to make sure the ice packs were in the freezer and my car was nearby. I became addicted to Sponge Bob and couldn't wait to cuddle on the couch with my son to watch reruns about Patrick the Starfish and Mr. Crabs. The thought of hanging out with the "girls" became secondary in my desire to be a better mother and to nurse my MS when it demanded attention.

For eleven years I self-injected Beta Seron, which limited my time "out on the town" and eliminated wearing bathing suits and shorts in the summer, unless I wanted to show off my assortment of lovely injection site bruises. Football season no longer held the appeal it once did when my enthusiasm for WVU waned in the shadow of walking from the parking lot to my seat, sweltering under the midday sun, stressing out over being the DD (since it wasn't convenient to "tail-gate" and do Beta Seron), and spending my entire day at the football stadium instead of taking advantage of those few hours in recovering for the work week ahead. I could no longer swim well, walk appropriately, go dancing, participate in aerobics class, tolerate a day of shopping, drive after dark (developing macular degeneration in one eye), or chase my child around the playground. I no longer wanted to be too far from home or risk the humiliation of public intoxication accusations.

If the critical public only knew the truth about MS. I often wake up feeling cheated of something I didn't even get a chance to partake in. It is no fun waking with the killer hangover headache that does its job expertly by hanging on ALL DAY LONG. No amount of water or ibuprofen can faze the sucker. My hands get shaky and I get a bit nauseated. My eyeballs even hurt and I swear I can feel the very core of my hair follicles. The light is excruciating, but I know this is not a migraine. Of course, my drop foot is more pronounced and I cannot trust myself to maneuver a car or even try to read the newspaper without shaking. The bugger about all of this is that I had not had even a faint inhale of alcohol to cause this.

But, this is just one day. Tomorrow will probably be different.

The point is…why does MS have this crazy effect on our bodies? Is it better to indulge in the very things that usually make us feel not so great afterward in order to fend off the ill effects of MS? Is this why some MSers use marijuana (legal, I hope) to ward off MS?

"Pot" has never been something that interested me. It has never given me the thrill that others seem to derive from its use. Even a very close family member has encouraged me to try the eatable version of marijuana because he says it will steady my nerves (really?) and help me venture into that nirvana state of "so what" in which I will forget my MS pains and enjoy life more fully. Well, sorry. I do not see feeling paranoid about my physical and mental condition as stress free. Besides, I do not have any pains I think marijuana is going to erase. But, what works for one doesn't always service another. Always remember that MS is a designer disease. It is a thumbprint. MS is extrememly personal.

So, back to the topic of this chapter. What other ailments do I experience on a day-to-day journey?

*My sinuses have always played a large role in my life. Right this very minute I am sniffling and snuffling and blowing my nose. It is year round and most common in the morning. It really becomes embarrassing when standing in front of my classroom and snot decides to run free- style down my face. Tissues are a must have.

*When I was still having my "monthly" I swear I experienced probably the WORST cramps known to womankind. NO joke. Complete with all the indecencies a gal could ever hope for. I will not go into detail here. Text me if you want to discuss the horrors of womanhood.

*My legs ache and have for years. I remember being quite young and begging my mother to rub my legs. Fifty-five years old and I still wish someone would perform this service for me. In fact, I find myself sometimes fantasizing about hiring a professional to give me a daily deep muscle foot and leg massage.

*Fatigue is a big one, but I have learned some tips on fighting that. Surprisingly one is to not over sleep. Periodic "catnaps" are wonderful, but not often fitting in to a work schedule. I understand this is not always feasible and I truly believe our country should think about adopting a more Mexican outlook on life. Why can we not have a national siesta rule? Working folks, students, full-time parents, medical personnel, coal miners...I cannot think of one individual who would not benefit from this. Just a little break around mid-day would serve us all well. And I suggest 2:00PM since that is when I know I definitely feel my body, mind, and mood curl up and say "goodnight."

So, maybe I am not as much fun or as interesting to be around as I once was, but I know my limitations. And, speaking of knowing about me...if folks stopped by more often, they might realize I probably accomplish more now than I ever did.

Ouch!

Just because I was diagnosed with an incurable disease doesn't make me any less Lisa. Sure, I might have a more serious attitude toward self-preservation than I once did, but I am still me. So, if you liked me prior to D Day, my inner self has not changed much.

I know conversing with someone with a disability (invisible or not) makes some people uncomfortable. What does one say? What does one suggest? My advice is when in doubt, don't mention MS. It doesn't have to be the focus of social conversation. In fact, I would rather it not be approached at all. I am not embarrassed by my condition (anymore), but I am truly embarrassed for those who feel they must address my health.

We all have (or soon will have) our own list of the most ridiculous/embarrassing MS-related comments. Here are some of mine:

You still have that (MS)?

When did you catch that disease?

You must really have it bad if you're still taking drugs.

Aren't you afraid your son will catch MS from you?

Oh, you've got one of those alphabet diseases. I can never keep them straight.

Didn't Lou Gehrig die from multiple sclerosis?

Why are you walking with a cane? (This from the same person who asks every time he sees me).

Oh, you probably wouldn't want to come (to whatever social event is being discussed). We'll probably be out late.

I thought you would outgrow it.

My neighbor had MS. He died last week.

Well, guess what? Yes, I still have MS. I plan to take it to the grave with me, but I do not plan to go to the grave because of it. And, I'm still a fairly interesting person. I go to sporting events. I drink beer. I read books and watch movies. I go shopping (if I must) and I prepare meals. I just do it more in moderation and I listen to my body.

Whoa, and someone had the nerve to say that Common Sense was dead?

Chapter Five

How 'Bout a HUG?

Spring Break 2014 Journal

This is my week in a nut shell—It's Spring Break (yes, we didn't get enough days out of school this year :) and my family normally spends a few days at our home away from home...Bemis, the Center of the Universe.

This year, however, I get to stay home for most of the week, entertaining doctors. For some time, I have suffered weird chest pains that were originally diagnosed as some kind of chest inflammation that required 3 daily doses of high power Motrin. It helped for a while but after several months I became nervous about the amount of Motrin that my body was ingesting...and the pain was not going away. So...I took my concerns back to the physician who has now decided that a pain pill (when needed) is more the ticket, in addition to a muscle relaxant at bedtime. It's done wonders, but a further precaution is the heart monitor that I am wearing for the next 24 hours. My heart rate is (I guess) alarmingly low, (Isn't that a good thing?) so I have been referred to a cardiologist and am proceeding with caution. I just hope that this new doctor journey does NOT interfere with WesTest. Oh, the complications that would create! (Seeing as how this educational measure of student achievement and teacher competency is more important than ANYTHING in my profession.)

(but I am anemic), but considering my family history I fully intend to see the cardiologist anyway. What's another day away from school if it assures me more days to enjoy my son? Westest, be damned. (Oops, did I really say that?)

So...I finally spent some of my break in the Center of the Universe, but it was short-lived. I felt horrible when I got there, went to bed early, and awoke even earlier...in tears. And I mean full blown hysteria. I could not stop crying, my chest hurt, my mind was imploding with terribly depressing images of anything and everything bad that could happen to me and to my family. I was so jittery I could barely dress myself. After a LONG, hot shower, I packed my things and drove home, scared behind words and unable to squelch my periodical bouts of crying. My poor son had to witness this and did his best to make me feel better. My baby is becoming such a wonderful young man. I told him to stay at camp with my husband, but he wanted to go with me just in case.

We drove immediately to my doctor, where I underwent another EKG and more blood work. The diagnosis? I have an ear infection, which was causing my dizziness. Better yet, the muscle relaxant was the main culprit. "Some people experience periods of depression." Lucky me, I'm one in that statistic.

The next day...

The antibiotic is working miracles. I am no longer dizzy or jittery. My chest pains are even gone.

I'm still going to the cardiologist, but I will NEVER take another muscle relaxant.

My son and I had a long talk about drug consumption. (Yep, forever the teacher in search of that "teachable" moment :) I am totally blown away by what that teeny, tiny little white pill did to me. In fact, I only consumed a fourth of it. He agrees that recreational drug use is NOT in his future. Good boy.

So…I am now on an essential oil kick. Noni juice has already proven its benefits regarding MS. Vitamin D is crucial. Peppermint always calms my tummy and there's nothing more relaxing than a hot cup of chamomile tea. Honey is an awesome natural remedy for many things. I'll keep my antibiotic for now, though.

My goal is to discover a good medical reason to eat all this yummy Easter chocolate in my kitchen.

Experiencing strange physical, mental, and emotional symptoms is all a part of life. So, I am thankful that I experienced that little Spring Break fiasco. It means I'm still kicking. Seriously, can you think of any Super Hero without his/her ultimate opponent?

After careful thought, I put Common Sense to work and did my best to get clinical about the situation. Both of my parents have had a heart attack, so I understand the concern with my heart health. Since that didn't seem to be my problem, my pal Common Sense waved his flag.

Have you ever heard of a hug gone wrong?

The MS Hug apparently is well-known to MSers. (Somehow I missed that memo.)

The MS Hug (also known as girdling) is a collaboration of symptoms caused by spasms in the intercostal region of the body. This is the area between the ribs. The Hug is often described as a squeezing, crushing, ants crawling under the skin, hot or cold burning, pins and needles sensation. Can we get any more vague in our attempt to be specific? That is just one example of how very custom-made MS presents itself. As no two snowflakes are alike, very few MS participants are identical.

I suffered with a diagnosis of a "floating rib" for thirteen years before realizing that my discomfort was most likely a MS Hug. After years of expensive chiropractor appointments and an excessive consumption of 800 milligram Ibuprofen, Common Sense tapped me (rather forcefully) on the shoulder and demanded that I remember my position in life. I have MS and I am a Super Hero. This in itself set me aside from the mainstream.

So, I added MS Hug to my arsenal of super powers and got busy fighting its ill effects. Two popular anti-spasticity muscle relaxants prescribed to ease the MS Hug are Baclofen and Diazepam.

I am more comfortable using a heating pad or scheduling a massage to ease my Hug discomfort. In fact, I sometimes just lie on the floor and stretch to find relief. We are all different.

So, find your inner snowflake and put your signature on your MS.

Chapter Six

"OWW!"

This morning I awoke with the same gluey eyes that greet me every morning. Between allergies, an overly active sinus condition, and macular degeneration in the left eye that plays with the cataract in the right eye, it is not surprising that my vision is not totally clear when I arise in the morning. But today it was different. Even after applying liquid tears and blinking to cover every nanno section of my eye balls, my eyesight was still incredibly fuzzy. I put on my eye glasses for reinforcement and found no improvement whatsoever. When I closed my left eye, I had a pretty good clear view with my right eye, but when I alternated this little exercise, my left eye absolutely refused to clear at all.

This just figured. My eye glass prescription changes yearly, if not more frequently, but I just acquired new glasses two weeks before in preparation for the new school year. My insurance would NOT agree to another eye exam so soon. And the deal I got on my new frames (the first I had had in several years because I thought it was just cheaper to continue recycling my old frames and replacing the lenses), would not repeat itself with the acquisition of pair number two. So, as I often do in life, I conceded to the fact that I just have to live with it. It is what it is.

But it sucks.

And this reminds me of a line in an original story by a young writer friend. I met Nick at my family reunion a few years ago. When he discovered that I am a veteran English teacher/published author, he was anxious for a professional response to his prose. (Yep, sometimes regular people are Super Heroes. And this had nothing to do with MS.) This occupational hazard is one that most often physicians, medical specialists or lawyers probably try to avoid in social settings. A veteran English teacher, I decided early in my career the perfect "buzz kill" is to announce my profession. Even having the most amazing time and enjoying the company of a variety of people who seem to be reciprocating the entertainment, knowing there is an English teacher in the house instantly puts everyone on guard of their words and storytelling. I have tried to assure everyone I know and who know me and what I do, that I am off the clock at the final bell of the day and that I do not pass judgment in any way on my adult counter parts, especially in social settings. But few believe me and I sometimes find it difficult to believe myself.

Anywho…Young Nick reverently approached me with his sheaves of lined paper and practically bowed with them at my feet before trotting off to partake of the reunion fun with an assortment of young cousins. I was worried that the nature of our weekend would distract from any serious critiquing I could offer; but his words shouted out at me from the very first line and I knew I had a talented young man awaiting any words of praise or encouragement I could offer.

I would not say that I had discovered the next Hemingway, but compared to students I have had in my nest, I honestly say this fella has a gift. I admire the honesty in his writing voice and hope that whatever guidance I can give him is worth the wait. The one line in his story that has not left me and haunts my thoughts is probably something that has been said repeatedly in his circle of acquaintances. I have probably overheard it in the hallways myself, but reading it over and over again struck me with a freshness I did not expect.

In his story, Nick writes in first person, the voice of my choice. He is a young male teen who is rather taken with a lovely young girl in his class and his attraction surprises him. I know from first-hand experience that young males of this age are often taken by storm when the hormones click in and they realize the opposite sex is rather fetching and there is something to be said about personal hygiene.

Anyway, the narrator has stunned himself with the realization he is even paying attention to this girl and once he peels his eyes off of her, he comments to himself, "It must suck to look so good."

(Dramatic Pause)

(Heavy sigh)

(Repeat previous directives.)

Think about it. "It must suck to look so good." There is nothing trivial about that comment. The honesty, the maturity of this statement is not typical of an eighth grade boy. The acceptance that all is not perfect in the world of popularity and good looks is not a trait common in this age group. If a girl is gorgeous and well-groomed, she must be: a) stuck up, b) a prep, c) a cheerleader with all the stereotypes that accompany that title, d) unapproachable. No one ever thinks about the consequences of beauty—especially at this young age.

Much like with having MS. Sure, we get the stares, we experience the avoidance and we silently endure the pains that plague us on a daily basis—but does the casual observer ever give this much thought? I mean, it does sound rather rude to approach a complete stranger, or even someone you know with these words, "Hey, man, it must suck to be you."

Wow. As MSers, we might think this to ourselves, but to actually verbalize it is way over the top. Even if it is true. We just do not do this. And yet, my new little writing friend nailed it without having a clue his words drove home a sentiment that encompasses the very being of practically every human being, regardless of age or gender.

It is such a shame that our MS symptoms and side-effects do not come with an absolute warning so that we can plan our daily events and life experiences around the inconveniences of the disease. It would be so very wonderful to at least be able to depend on a fair indication of an exacerbation or annoying symptom so that our social and professional calendars ran more smoothly.

Hell, yeah, it does suck being me. It sucks to have diabetes. It sucks to have a brain tumor. It sucks looking good. It sucks being bitten by a smart-ass parrot.

My brother's girlfriend has a talking bird that often gives him all the parrot love that she is capable of, rubbing affectionately against him, perching on his shoulder, or staring adoringly on to his face. When they first became acquainted he fell under her spell and didn't realize her attention was a false sense of security in her devotion. After a few "bird attacks" his attraction to her waned drastically and Abby (the bird, not the girlfriend) was relegated to her cage when he was in the room.

He learned there is nothing as painful as being bitten by an irate parrot. But then, he started paying close attention to the bird's behavior when he was around. Abby really did seem to like him and approve of his relationship with her "master," but he noticed when she tired of his human sentiments, she would emit a little squawk and pronounce quite clearly, "Oww," before offering her extremely painful bite.

Though the bird does not speak the Queen's English, nor does she communicate as her human counterparts do, she obviously related a very human sentiment with a related action. And she let her prey know what was to come.

I hate it when I find myself unexpectedly kissing the floor or unsuccessfully forcing my legs to obey a desperate plea to MOVE. My MS does not warn me of these surprise parties by saying, "Oww," or creating mental red flags before organizing a full blown attack. Sometimes I do not even feel the "bite" until I am already inconvenienced by its war strategy. I wouldn't even mind borrowing this verbal feather friend if I thought she could warn me with her irony.

I know there are several things that I can avoid in order to subsequently avoid the ill results of MS, but that isn't the same thing. Staying out of the heat is a smart move. Getting plenty of rest and fitting in some time to exercise are good things. Eliminating stressful situations and negative relationships are very, very good ideas as well; but with MS, it is not always that easy. And MS does not give us a variety of choices.

We can choose to diet or exercise. We can decide whether or not to plan a day around work or fun. It is our human ability to stop smoking, read a book, watch a movie, buy a new dress, or indulge in self-serving activity or volunteer for a community project. We do not get to choose with MS. MS is in the driver's seat and gets to make most of the decisions in everyday life. MS is full of "Oww" moments, the majority of which come with no forewarning.

Of course, life does not come equipped with clear cut cautions, so we must spend some time to analyze the cause and effect of life.

I have an uncle who lost his leg to diabetes and is finding it very difficult emotionally, as well as physically, in adapting his life around the loss of mobility and independence. There were many warnings in his life about the possibility of such a tragedy and often he really did have control over the consequences of his life choices.

When living with any disease, we need to know our limitations. I am not saying he choose to lose a limb, but there are always choices that can help us guard against such consequences. Maybe his lifestyle dictated the turn his unfortunate disease developed. Maybe he just didn't pay attention to those OW moments.

I mentioned my Parrot Brother, but there is a second sibling in my family. My other brother fell victim to a brain tumor several years ago. He had always suffered headaches that increasingly became more and more painful and frequent over the years, but were never connected with the possibility of this tumor. They were probably early signs of his condition, but headaches are not always viewed as cause to consider a brain disease. They are more commonly considered an inconvenience and annoying part of life. They might have been his "Oww," but he didn't know that.

After three brain surgeries, the tumor is mostly removed. There is no cancer and he has successfully regained most of his bodily functions. I often think it is rather strange that he and I share many of the same neurological symptoms although our conditions are not the same. Or, are they? His tumor and my MS are both conditions of the brain. The right side of his body suffers the most, as does mine. We both limp around and favor our right legs. The biggest difference, other than the obvious diagnosis, is that he prefers and tolerates heat while I definitely demand cooler temperatures. I find it a little weird how our brains are conditioned to these differences in order to properly function within the boundaries of our physical conditions.

Neurology is neurology, I guess. It is all an "Oww" attack.

There is really not much we can do about it, but we can learn to know ourselves.

I miss a lot of social events since recognizing and appreciating the warnings of my body. Sure, a lot of it is intuition, but it makes sense. I do not put myself in any situation that I know I cannot escape. I try to always sit near a door and at the end of a row in movie theaters, church, and meetings. This assists my mobility and eliminates any imposition on other folks around me.

I must always know the location of the ladies room and I plan any outing around the floorplan of the space around me. I don't even shop in grocery stores if I don't know where the restroom is because I invariably must "go" as soon as I enter the store.

I have always preferred to be on the front row, closest to the action, but not anymore. I have sacrificed my straight-A mentality in order to accommodate the MonSter. You know what they say— Keep your friends close and your enemies closer. Common Sense is my right-hand pal, but the MonSter is always in my sight.

Chapter Seven

The Flop Drop

While researching my most annoying symptom of MS, I had to giggle when I found this most apt description of my malady. Flop Drop. That really does sum it up.

My foot literally "flops" when it is not in a communicative mood. It actually sounds rather disgusting, but it is such a more literal and accurate description of this common MS trait.

I hate it when I am feeling particularly peppy, but my right foot decides to rebel, leaving me left behind in more ways than one. It is one horrible thing to feel my age when my mind is still programed to partake in all things young and active, but when my body just refuses to play the game because it cannot, I feel even more incapable of existing successfully in the human race.

Foot drop, or drop foot, is a common symptom of multiple sclerosis. It's a difficulty in lifting the front part of the foot, which can make walking a challenge. People with this symptom tend to walk by lifting the knee as though they were walking up stairs. I discovered that I suffer from drop foot after a series of stumbling, lurching, frightening falls that left me totally unnerved and rather depressed, as well as thoroughly embarrassed by the reactions of my friends. Of course, they thought I was drunk. I was doing the perfect imitation of the wino down the street.

I realized that was not the case when I ended up in the emergency room with an ugly gash in my forehead and a shiny black eye, following an unexpected fall one evening that I do not even remember. The last thing I remember was that I turned from one person to reply to someone else behind me and boom, I was on the ground. The corner of my eye was imbedded in the corner of a metal heat vent and I could not move my legs or arms to right myself. I do not know what happened. They do not know what happened.

I DO know and remember well that someone called my (ex) husband. The nightmare image of him standing across the room with my nine month old son in his arms, blatantly casting judgment over me and telling my friends to call an ambulance because I was in no condition for him to take to the hospital. My stomach twists still today as I remember my baby seeing his mother lying on the ground while his father mentally assured him that I was unfit and would most likely be removed from his life as soon as possible. (This is my former spouse.)

In my young adult novel, *Abby*, the main character relays an incident in the grocery store parking lot when her mother (recently diagnosed with MS) is cited by an ignorant bystander as being drunk and totally irresponsible for involving her own children in her public display of inappropriateness. Abigail is appalled, embarrassed, and anxious that her mother overheard the offensive remarks.

I, too, worry about the reactions of other people when they see me stumble along a perfectly clear and level walkway. It is even worse when I am accompanied by my own son, husband (current and forever spouse), or other innocent escort. It is one thing to belittle me, but I take total offense when people I care about have to suffer the shame of knowing me. It is not fair to them. My companions didn't ask to be associated with such a derelict.

The up side of this, though, is the creation of such labels as the Flop Drop. I mean, really. How can one even say this without giggling? MS is not funny. There is nothing amusing about "flopping" around, but the best way to cope with MS is with some inside humor. Folks in "the know" understand our need for little inside jokes like this.

Just call me an over achiever, but I have experimented with a variety of drop foot eliminators including one of those wire-controlled devices designed to eliminate drop foot through electronic stimulus. I think it is probably a wonderful tool for folks who can afford it or whose insurance recognizes it as a viable treatment for MSers. Mine, unfortunately, does not; but, I could diverse very quickly onto the topic of what the "real" world views as important.

We have all experienced this. Because we cannot understand MS and because it cannot be categorized in black and white terms as far as definition, there is no true documentation to make it a "real" disease, so funding for this imaginary condition is not justified with the powers who hold the purse strings. Whoops!

Showing my cynical persona.

Sorry.

Deep sigh.

It's me.

I'm back: Miss Positive.

I have discovered several alternatives to the expensive, manu-factured suggestions. The problem with drop foot and properly fit-ting shoes seems to be with how the foot is positioned within the confines of the shoe. You can actually rig a small bungee cord attach-ment in the shoe that forces the front of the foot to lift at the appropri-ate time when taking a step.

This Flop Drop thingy sounds like an interesting and affordable idea. Sure, it's another money maker for some enthusiastic inventor, but some of mankind's best ideas have evolved from unexpected activities. (Who would have thought that flying a kite would start this whole electricity fad?)

After closely analyzing this Flop Drop device, I think I under-stand the physics of it. At first, I thought I could probably rig a similar doohicky (West Virginia slang for thingy, thingamajig, whatchamacallit), without the 'professional' accessorizing I am certain this factory-made tool includes. As far as I can tell, the most important part of the Flop Drop tool is the tiny bungee cord that seems to control the entire process.

Because I am just not crafty enough to put something like this together, I try to remember to do some leg lifts while sitting on the couch. Walking in place for ten minutes or more often helps, as long as you concentrate on lifting the heel, which forces the front of the foot to elevate.

My favorite footwear needs to fit securely to the foot and not slip up and down on the heel. Clark is my go-to brand, but can be pricey. I look for a bargain and when I find it, I wear the soles off my purchase. Flipflops just do not work for me and even the hint of a high heel is absolutely a no-go. I like boots in the fall and winter months and a comfy sneaker, securely laced, is good year 'round.

Okay, quit snooping my closet. If you want to know more about flop drop, check out this website. http://dropfootorthotics.com/learn-more/

Chapter Eight

Namaste, Y'all!

According to Multiple Sclerosis for DUMMIES (page 179), at one time, not long ago, people with MS were told "not to exercise." Of course only seventy-five years ago people with MS were also locked up in a psyche ward or hidden from society's prying eyes.

On the same page in MSFD (my own little acronym for the book I reference often), the authors offer a list of exercise benefits. It reduces fatigue, increases endurance and flexibility, improves cardiovascular health, improves bowel and bladder functions, strengthens bones, improves your mood, and helps in maintaining weight management. Okay, I don't think I plagiarized too blatantly. In a nutshell, exercise is good stuff and not just for people with MS. (Hello, Common Sense!)

I have played around with all types of exercise all of my life and when MS presented its own challenge to me, I realized that my exercise regime needed to take a serious turn from high impact aerobics to more manageable options.

"Yoga!" the specialists urge.

"Yes, yoga!" my neurologist choruses.

"Yoga is the thing!" all of my research indicates.

"Namaste," my cat's wise eyes tell me.

My first gentle yoga session was with New York guru Charles on my Yoga Zone DVD. As he led me through the various poses on the "sun drenched beaches" of his location shoot in Jamaica, I felt rather deflated at the lack of aerobic involvement. I silently (not to insult the cat) resolved to use this as my daily stretching routine before I jumped on my stationary bicycle for a two or three mile ride.

Ha, ha, ha, ha, ha, ha!

Lesson learned: Yoga is NOT for sissies.

When I flopped to the floor on day two of this yoga commitment (and, flopped I did because for some reason my leg muscles refused to flow as fluidly as the day before) I realized what Charles and I had done hours before had literally "touched a nerve." Behind his sweet smile and his calm voice was a task master whose sword was drawn in defense against the MonSter. And, so, I answered his challenge and held a daily twenty minute rendezvous with Charles for several weeks. And, as Allen Finger (the founder of Yoga Zone and fleeting narrator of my DVD) asserts, this is "the workout that will change your life."

At the end of week one, I was already feeling the positive effects of yoga. I subscribed to Yoga Magazine and actually purchased a yoga mat. I was on my way to becoming a Yogi. I had visions of long weekend retreats in remote areas of the country, sipping whole fruit juice concoctions while listening to the hypnotic meditations of Charles and his fellow Yogis.

At this point, I felt confident in my yoga practice. I was ready to explore other instructors and make more Yogi friends. (That's the way with MS. It often forces us into a reclusive lifestyle where our friends are DVD actors and television personalities. MS is a jealous companion and wants you all to itself.)

I realized that I was doing more observing than actual participating when I tuned in to Sadie Nardini (Rock Your Yoga) on the Veria channel. Sure, I stretched, I rocked, I admired her interesting collection of Yoga wear. I did whatever I was told until it became too challenging for me to continue. When this happened, I just folded into a child's pose and thought about what I should do with my day.

I was missing a most important message. When the practicing yogis tell you that child's pose is always "there for you," they mean to assume child's pose until your breath settles and you are ready to move on with your practice. They do NOT mean you have completed your yoga session for the day. Child's Pose is a resting place, not the conclusion to your yoga session. I needed an expert to drive this home before I truly understood. Because I really, really, love Child's Pose.

Through the National Multiple Sclerosis Society I discovered MYMSYOGA with Baron Baptiste and Dr. Elliot Frohman. This is a free DVD offered by NMSS and has enlightened me that my yoga practice has not been doing me any justice. When I play with my yoga tapes, I am not practicing with yogis purposefully directing an audience of particularly situated individuals. After working with my new DVD for several days (No, I could not make it entirely through the entire DVD the first day.), I realized that Baron is not watering down his practice to fit my physical condition. (And I started on the Foundation level!) What he does, though, is constantly reassure his viewers that it is okay to "fall out" of a pose. It is acceptable to feel unstable and to remember that child's pose is there for you...as a resting place...for a minute or two...not for the entirety of the class.

I like that the participants in his recorded sessions are a variety of age, gender, and physicalities. I can relate to at least one woman as obviously having a drop foot or similar affliction that forces her to pay special attention to that leg.

A drop foot is often "left behind" in physical situations. I cannot forcibly lift or raise my right foot in order to put on my pants or even to bring it to a reclining position without assisting it with my hands. Sucks, yep! Because I realize now I have basically enabled my right leg to collect welfare instead of working a steady shift, I have a lot of work to do to make it work for me now. Thirty minutes with Baron and you will discover that as well.

It took me some time before moving on to Baron Baptiste's second level, "Transformations," and I admittedly am frightened of the third and final level. And, that's okay. Even Allen Finger would agree that this Yoga journey is a patient pursuit. In yoga we are urged to be "ever mindful" in our practice, because that is an essential part of this activity. Living with MS is a practice in being ever mindful of everything we do.

Living with MS requires planning and careful decision making. We do not simply leap into an activity, even if that activity is as simple as preparing breakfast. We MSers must take time and thought into consideration for every single thing we do.

I recommend Yoga, but it is not the only feasible alternative to channel surfing. My son's Wii has proven invaluable to me. Wii Fit Plus offers an excellent assortment of movement options, as does Weight Watchers DVD series. And that's what it is all about—movement.

It doesn't matter if you exercise in the privacy of your own home or in a structured public environment. Just Move!

Water aerobics is highly recommended as well. The buoyancy of working out in the water is so much kinder to the joints and just makes movement easier. But, it's a public activity and one that requires showing off that bikini bod. But, that's okay because generally the participants are concentrating on the class and not each other.

My advice: Find an activity that you enjoy and just MOVE!

Namaste.

Chapter Nine

Comments From the Crowd

This disease is getting more and more populated every day. The more I read, the more I study, the more I just observe everyday life, the more I find that MS is no longer the catch-all for any and every unidentified medical condition. MS has simply become more recognizable. And that is good. For us, not for MS. (Remember: MS is the Bad Guy. WE are the Super Heroes).

Did you know that just a few years ago, in the 1950s, people with what was later identified as MS were actually institutionalized for their random symptoms of uncontrolled body functions, slurred speech, unsteady gait and inability to freely care for themselves? We were considered freaks, oddities, natures' jokes on an otherwise well-ordered society. We were locked away from view and often times not even given the respect of an examination.

It is human nature to fear that which we do not understand. Well, guess what? I do not understand trigonometry, but I am not afraid of it. It may not be on my list of most comfortable subjects, but I am determined not to let it to keep me awake at night.

MS sometimes DOES keep me up at night, but I am no longer afraid of it. I want to understand it, but I am intelligent enough to realize that sometimes there are those entities in life that are not meant to be understood. I hate the axiom, "live with it," but that is also the best advice to offer when all other remedies have been exhausted. I do not mean to imply we no longer have a responsibility to learn as much as possible about this disease and we should jump off the train of support.

But sometimes we just have to take responsibility for our own selves. You have surely seen the announcement that Common Sense has died? The obituary used to be posted in our teacher's lounge at school. SOAP BOX SPOILER: Society does not seem to feel that we are responsible for our own actions any more. We are the victim. We have no control. Bullshit.

You heard me.

Bull.

Shit.

Common Sense is my partner in crime. Robin to my Batman.

I know when I do not feel well. I am aware of what brings me pain and what I can do to forestall or even eliminate that pain. Of course, I am a pride freak, too. MY biggest handicap is that I do not like to be at the mercy of someone else when I am capable of taking care of myself. I have learned, though, to rely on people when they volunteer and to not feel shame for it. If I fall, I find a way to climb back on my feet. If I need assistance, I ask for it. (And then I find a quiet place to shed my tears of physical pain, humiliation or frustration.) I get on with it. I avoid as much undo attention as possible. But, I guess that's just me.

Having MS is a full-time job. And it's hard work!

Thus, having MS requires Super Human powers. And A LOT of interaction with your support group.

After nearly 15 years battling the MonSter, I am finally figuring out how to sort through the kryptonite. Support groups come in all shapes and sizes. Upon initial diagnosis, I was encouraged to actually join a physical MS support group. I did, but it was too soon for me. Although I was greeted with open and loving arms, the reality of my situation crashed around me with dread. The president of the county Blue Ridge MS Group is one of the sweetest people ever. Her concern over my recent diagnosis was evident. And she was sincere.

But she scared me.

As did a former colleague, who bowed quietly over her wheel chair lap tray as her husband fed her the pretty snacks arranged on a side bar in the bright hotel conference room.

And there was the brother of one of my dearest friends, whose sister also had been introduced to the MonSter several years before. Both of his walking sticks (one for each hand) rested neatly against the table where he sat alone.

Probably the most frightening member of this group was the one who appeared the most normal. "Jen" was a young mother of two. She literally bounced around the room, pony tail flying, dong her best to greet every one and monopolize individual conversations. Her excitement over the arrival of someone new to the program and possibly closer to her own age was a visible cloud that followed her movements.

Beneath all that excitement to be there, beneath the wall of her cheerful words and sincerely interested questions, hidden behind those bright eyes…I saw FEAR.

And that FEAR raced through the air to lodge itself in the exposed nerve endings of my own dying myelin. (Okay, that is rather over the top. But, my inner Super Hero was in its infancy.)

By the conclusion of the meeting, Jen was bouncing up and down in her seat between my mother and me, anxiously holding out a post-it note that held her phone number and home address.

We were to be 'besties' for all time.

I haven't returned to Support Group and often feel very guilty about that. I really do intend to revisit sometime and I hope I find the welcome just as inviting and the spirits as hopeful. In this time of social media, I am more comfortable in front of my computer conversing with the masses all at once. Face Book is awesome as long as you are wary of the allure to predators.

My go-to Face Book support page is, We're Not Drunk, We Have MS. The folks there are extremely forthright in their approach to this MonSter we share. I do not contribute much online, but I enjoy the comradery. (I'm a Lurker.) The dialogue I have witnessed exhibits an honest and sincere concern for the members. When I

But...I will dwell on that later. My main focus right now is to endure the next twenty-four hours so I can get ready for my planned Spring Break.

I'm not worried about the heart monitor and I actually appreciate the fact I have to avoid using the telephone or the microwave while wired to this gadget. I find public interest in this visual indication of an infliction fascinating, though. Just because the little black box and accompanying gray wires are part of my attire today, complete strangers are compelled to sympathetically comment on my "situation." It doesn't hurt that my drop foot is acting up today so my gait is a bit "off." For nearly thirteen years I have evidently passed off my MS as just an annoyance, rather than a daily complication. Now, because I am connected to a physical reminder of a possible "condition," my fellow Earth occupants dig into their generosity banks to offer encouraging words. Hmmm.....

I try not to call attention to my MS and mostly do a pretty good job of that. I have been using my cane more often of late and that has produced questions, especially from my students since I don't really go anywhere else but school. Two comments in the last week, one from a student and one from a colleague, "Mrs. McCombs, what's with the cane?"

"Oh, my. How did you hurt your ankle?"

When I admit my MS, I do not do so with shame, and I do not mind offering an abbreviated description of the disease. I just hate admitting to a weakness, regardless of the fact that it is nothing I caused. It is humiliating enough that I need to justify my physical limitations, but the confusion exhibited by an onlooker is sometimes even worse.

Five Days Later

Ah...but it gets better..

The heart monitor was no big deal and all test results are encouraging. There is supposedly nothing wrong with my heart asked for assistance in completing this chapter in my book, the response was overwhelming.

I posted this request:

To complete a current research "project," I need to compile a list of the biggest MS complaints. If you would like to help, please tell me your "kryptonite."

Stress
Heat
Bladder
Heat
Over-stimulation...visual, audio, mental....sensory overload I would
    call it
Heat
Heat + humidity
Fatigue
Blindness
Over stimulation, definitely!!!!
HEAT and HUMIDITY
Back Pain and cognitive issues
Heat, cold
Stress and humidity
Heat and stress.
Stress
Heat, over stimulation, bowel and bladder. Fatigue, insomnia
Fatigue
Balance/walking and bowel incontinence are most embarrassing
Bladder
Weakness, balance,walking
Pain and no energy...oh and bowel issues...I hate that!!!!!
    PAIN!!!!!!!!! balance/walking! Vertigo, cold, fatigue and stress
Not having the stamina/energy to do what I once did. This brings
    on severe depression for me.
Heat, fatigue, foot drop, bowel and bladder urgency. LOL but I
    have had MS for 30 years so it's my new normal. I just symp-

tom manage based on the weather, my strength, and what can be accomplished that day or sometimes within an hour. Good luck! I miss school soooooooo much! I dreamed of law school and becoming a criminal defense lawyer. xoxo

Fatigue, stress and heat for me smile emoticon

Heat - from outside or even the shower, get it a bit warm in the morning and I MUST GO BACK TO BED.

Humidity....and headaches from my eyes straining to see....makes me want to rip my eyeball out

Hug, Fatigue PAIN that feels like toothache.

Vertigo, numbness in my hands, MS hugs in abdominal area, lower immune systems mean longer heal time and easier to catch colds. Use of canes and walkers for balance. Tons of different meds to control different symptoms.

STRESS!!!!

MS Hug

Heat.

Stress.

Heat, cold, noise, fatigue, no appetite, balance, bladder, constipation, insomnia, numbness, memory, concentration.

Heat intolerance, Memory loss

Attention span, gone.

Fatigue and heat

Weakness,numbness on left side of body,heat,fatigue,balance,trouble walking and stress

Fatigue

Unable to think clearly or remember information.

Thought process unable to get what I want to say out.

I miss running and walking the dogs

Cognitive problems!! Fatigue and stress

Fatigue

Energy and headaches Brain Farts to me are awful.

Walking. Unable to feel my feet and right side. Pain. Spasms in right foot and leg. Speech is slurred. Double vision in both eyes and sight very poor in right eye. Fatigue most of time. Bladder problems. Laugh when I shouldn't. Memory loss. Unable to sleep. I'm sorry you just wanted one.

Short term memory is shot after almost 20 years! Off ALL DMDs! old intolerance!

Fatigue and major major short and long term memory loss.

Fatigue.

Fatigue!!! Hands and feet numbness and tingling. Heat and cold intolerance.

Walking, is my biggest complaint

WALKING!

I get really weird symptoms, like right now the big toe on my right foot feels broken, this is not the first time for my toes to feel this way on either foot.

Walking.

Heat HEAT HEATTTT, and or lack of sleep (with newborns)

Bladder issues.

Fatigue

Heat + MS = fatigue

Humidity /Heat

Heat

You are the first one to say that about the toe, makes me feel better that I am not the only one with that strange symptom!

The heat!

Heat-fatigue

Heat/fatigue/bladder issues

Cognitive problems.

The heat which makes the fatigue much worse and the sweating which causes me to be unable to do normal activities.

Short term memory loss, numbness in hands and fingers, weak knees

Cognition, balance/stairs and fatigie.

Heat and doctors that do not believe that there is pain associated with MS

Heat intolerance. Cog fog. Fatigue.

Leg pain which affects walking. I still drive enough to more than get by. I don't use a cane or walking aids on daily basis just motorized carts at stores. Bladder/bowel issues rank really high because of inconvenience.

Heat. It brings everything on. Fatigue, walking difficulty, cognitive disfunction, numbness and tingling, weakness, etc. Depending on what the flavor of the day is.

feeling inadequate!!!

Ms hug/costocondritis, had some chest pain daily since Jan 2.

Interrupted speech, brought on by anger, stuttering, etc, heat intolerance, loss of use of left hand because of numbness, dropping everything I hold onto. Dropped foot, causing dragging and constant stubbing of toe!

Being tired ALL THE TIME.

There's a couple of issues but for me the one that gets me the most is memory issues.

heat intollarence, I wilt in direct sunlight

Leg drop, legs dragging

Hot weather causes major fatigue,along with seizures if i become over heated. Cold weather brings increase of pain.

Heat - can be a fever or the weather

Heat sensitivities number one... stinging pricking feeling numbness in hands and feet #2... fatigue #3..feeling that im going to faint #4. Head feeing weird brain fog with blurred dimmed vision #5 leg pains and throbbing sensation comes in at a close 6.. And being in the cold brings about worsening of these symptoms. Lastly bladder spams along with urgency of having to urinate continually and anxiety attacks.

Heat fatigue memory swallowing problems numbness body temperature changes

Overheating is definately my kryptonite. My brain fries, I am feeling as though my body is burning from the inside out. Icepacks applied to my legs and body and neck and arms melts rapidly.

The heat is the same for me.

Stress

Tired all the time, I sleep more than I'm awake

Bladder problems

Fatigue

Bladder!

Stiffness and cognitive along with balance.

Vison issues and how it impacts my driving / not being able to drive at night.

Baccafin took my legs away

The belief from others there isn't pain w ms.. no pain my foot!

Balance

Balance, foot drop,

balance and right frozen fingers.

Heat/resultant cramping.

Heat! causes paresthesia.itching,burning of skin

Walking / balance issues for sure.... heavy legs, foot drop

Walking/balance problems, loss of my bladder

Heat, balance and not being able to poop on a normal schedule

My biggest complaint is that my right leg is very weak. I am still walking - with a Walkaide and a cane. It is a struggle.

HUMIDITY!! It suffocates me, tightens my body beyond comfort emotionally wants to put me in a place I don't want to be in and I fight it even when I try to ignore it

My balance is very poor, heat affects me most

Lisa McCombs—Wow! You folks are the best. I am currently writing a common sense book to dealing with the MonSter and really needed some practical input from fellow MSers. This is fantastic.

Tireness all the time balance issues memory issues sniffness heat and cold intolerance pain all over weakness in legs arms trouble sleeping wake up soaking wet.

My biggest two are HEAT and stress. I absolutely hate summer. If I get hot I get so weak and shakey I feel like I'm going to faint. And I can't do anything to stop or help it except stay cool. The stress issue is something I just have to be careful about and figure ways to relax. Easier said then done sometimes but necessary. Yes, you can quote me. Let me know if I can be of any more help.

Fatigue and heat.

Balance and weak legs are a big problem. It keeps me from driving. Remembering anything is very hard. Sometimes I have to read a paragraph 2 or3 times before I can remember it and continue.

Phantom itching ...

Fatigue! See Translation

Drop foot. Feels like someone has my foot in a vice a large majority of every day. Spasticity also very bad in one leg.

Other people!!

Slightly off track, semantics,doctors saying there is no "pain" associated with MS

Weakness in legs and leg spasms

Drop foot and uncontrollable spasticity at night

Fatigue and cold

Pain, Fatigue, Depression.

Unable to remember anythig

Visual disturbances

Depression

Fear.

Right now the heat and humidity, stuck in house 24/7 and hate missing the summer by being in the house. But if I go out at all I get so weak I will fall down and the pain will go thru the roof.

heat and overdoing things is my worst

PAIN! In my legs and most recently arms, The MS hug wich is an awful name, and almost the worst my brain cognitive forget tons, can't learn new things don't remember people. I don't like too drive cause I always forget where I'm going and sometimes forget where I am and have to pull over.

Heat heat heat. And balance. But the heat wears me out.

HEAT.

Heat and Cold

Heat and Humidity def balance too, fatigue has to be my #1, but heat gets me to that point quicker

Crumbling teeth, fatigue, and pain

Peripheral nerve damage makes me itchy 24/7. sometime I cut my self when I scratch.

Lisa McCombs—I've not heard of the crumbling teeth; but that may explain why I keep chipping mine.

Uhtoff's phenomenon - heat is one of our worst enemies. Having to always have a "cooling off" plan can be burdensome, as well as the bulky, wardrobe fail (lol) of a cooling vest.

Fatigue and pain in head and face (kind of like lightening bolts)

Also, (one of) my (many) kryptonite is always hiding. Hiding the pain. Hiding the fatigue, hiding symptoms and saying "I am okay." This is so I am not always a "Debbie downer" so people won't mind being around me. Family drama.

HEAT!!! It causes so much damn depression that I cannot even get to Walmart without getting sick! The burning sensation in my pelvis and my legs, andTREMORS!!

Humidity & stress. (Aka hiding how I really feel & doing too much just to prove I'm not a useless lump!)

Wages Fatigue and heat.

Fatique and nerve pain

Pain, cog fog, and fatigue!

Heat, humidity and isolation/loneliness

Stress and gluten.

Like many of you fighting the heat and humidity, which is causing increased fatigue, and pain. I'm sooooo sick if being inside to deal with it!! But I have the same problems with the humidity in the cold. ughhh!!

Heat, humidity, depression

Heat. Cold. Stairs. Depression. Memory loss. Unable to open food without aid of scissors or kids. Migraine over a year. Sleep too much.

Pain, heat and fatigue

Fatigue, nerve pain, humidity, depression

Heat, depression, memory loss

Fatigue

Heat, FATIGUE, weakness, numbness, memory issues, etc. etc., etc.

"you don't look sick"

Fatigue

memory issues & uneducated people who make comments
Poor balance in
Loss of appetite
Fatigue, weakness, cognitive issues, bladder issues, PAIN, &
   MORE
Fatigue and heat
Fatigue
A messed up brain - no short term memory, forget everything I am
   supposed to do, can't do it right anymore.
Heat
Heat
Pain, heat, fatigue, stress
Fatigue and stress
Fatigue
Heat, seizures, vision
Stress and heat

*Lisa McCombs I am overwhelmed by the response my simple
   little request evoked! This is the first time since my diagnosis
   that I have ever been surrounded by so many folks who,
   literally, feel my pain. Please message me if you are not
   comfortable with your response being published. I will erase
   all the names from this post and only print your responses.
   But don't stop responding! I want to hear from all of you!*

Heat
Heat, stress & Cog Fog.
Stress is another huge one, it's like the silent exacerbator
What, can no one see it? smile emoticon My big pain is a loss of
   memory. I have the other things mentioned, but forgetting my
   son's names...it is horrible. Why can't I remember my son's
   names? It is a tough sentence. I use pet names, that helps
   sometimes.
Heat, fatigue, stress, and speech issues. Oh and tremors when I'm
   trying to do something with my hands.
My Pop didn't have MS and he could never remember any of his
   5 kids name sometimes. What you describe is pretty across the

board, unless you can't remember for 10 minutes or so....

Bladder/bowel incontinence, Heat, Fatigue, A LOT of Pain, Balance, Dizziness, Numbness, Muscle Spasms and of course uneducated, ignorant family/friends and society in general making comments about how we're not sick, that we are just seeking attention and drugs, all because we look fine on the outside!!

Dizziness/balance, permanent double vision

Heat. Stress. Latin men

Fatigue, dizziness, temperature intolerance

Foot drop

Memory/concentration. Forgot to put that in the first post. Lol

Balance and pain#1. Optic neuritis and damage trying to take right eye. Total hearing in right ear and specialist its permanent. Bladder, so many broken bones and falls. Now having swallowing issues, which is scary.

This time of year I have to say heat/humidity, but in the winter, cold really gets me as well. So for me, it's temps to far out of the comfort zone either way.

humidity being so high that in the heat I turn into a wet sponge, and cold weather slows me to a crawl. spacticity and pain

I like the months that are right in the middle wink emoticon

Steps, or walking up a moderately steep slope - turns my legs to jello everytime. But, so grateful to be able to walk.

Stress

Fatigue , stress, pain, dizziness, numbness those are what bothers me the most .... oopps there's another I almost forgot ... insomnia!! lol

Heat & memory

Muscle spasms

Walking/standing, Heat/humidity, other illnesses, bathroom issues, trying to multitask...nervous pressure.

Heat.

Fatigue

All of the above

Fatigue

Fatigue, heat and memory are my biggest issues amongst others...
Aches, fatigue
Fatigue and missing not being able to walk
Not being able to walk
Heat, fatigue, walking
Walking and balance
Balance & Heat
Depression
Humidity!
Heat and walking like I am drunk!
Heat and balance...
The numbness and tingling that is constant in my feet and legs
Not being able to walk
Heat
Walking and balance
Weakness, Fatigue and Balance
Also cognitive issues, mentioned above. I'm so lost in my own head that I don't really know or seem to care much about the world around me. I do, I'm just lost in my own head and it sucks. I'd talk to people more but I'm afraid that I'll sound worse because I'm so confused. Balance is shot, I hold on to things when I walk, but I'm thankful that I can still walk! (small victories)
"Penis numbness" If I get that permanently, just damn kill me, lol
Fatigue and heat.
Sexual dysfunction
Heat. Drop foot. And being tired
Humidity!!!
My worst issues are with changes in temp and memory and mentality...and foot drop and...
All of the above......minus the penis problems...
Heat, fatigue, walking
Memory, fatigue and insomnia
Heat, fatigue and anxiety/depression
humidity, extreme cold and insomnia
Heat and high humidity, stiff and painful legs, balance
Finding Doctors that truly understand

Stiffness and pain in legs ,Heat ,memory problems and many more
I know I,m forgetting
All the above, and not being able to sit on the floor to play toys
with my son
At this particular moment, the HEAT!!... Was outside for less than
15 mins and now my legs and feet are killing me and I feel dizzy,
like I'm about to pass out!!... The fan isn't even cooling me off
right now....
The heat affects me badly too, but it's winter here so at least I
don't have to deal with that right now.
This heat is killing my MS!! I put on my makeup, I don't know
why, it's gonna melt off!! Heading to dinner with friends, MS
you are not invited!!!

—Members of We're Not Drunk.
We Have MS! Facebook page.

These folks pretty much wrote this chapter for me. If you weren't a believer prior to reading this, there is something not quite human about you if you don't believe now.

Lesson learned?

No, matter where you are in your disease, know that you are not alone. And you do not need to be alone.

Know your kryptonite. Be armed and face the enemy with an attitude.

Yes, we have MS, but we are armed and dangerous!

We are everywhere.

We are warriors.

We are Super Heroes.

Chapter Ten

Is it hot enough for ya?

Talk about the perfect day for a football game! September 3, 2004, promised to be a stellar day to be outside and to be a Mountaineer fan.

I dressed for the promised heat and was happy to wear my newest WVU shirt in celebration of opening day. I had decaled my fingernails with flying WVUs the night before and made certain to wear the perfect pair of Mountaineer earrings to match my corresponding bracelet. My latest splurge was a pair of blue and gold trimmed New Balance tennis shoes.

It wasn't only a ballgame day. Oh, no. I had a date for that football game.

For the first time since my diagnosis, I was going to enjoy a day without worrying about my disease or the ill effects MS plays on other people in my life. My two and a half year old son was with his Grammy and today was my opportunity to remember how it feels to have a social life.

I know that sounds selfish and thoroughly self-serving, but I had been a very, very good girl since my divorce. I hadn't thought about dating or having any type of relationship other than the one I had enjoyed with my son. I tell him often that he saved my life. That, if not for him, I do not really know what would have become of me after discovering my disease. With him to care for, I had a purpose for plunging ahead, for staying involved in life, for wanting to enjoy my job, my church, and my life.

That is not to say that I did not miss having a little adult fun from time to time.

My date was an old friend from the past and a colleague in the recent realm of divorcehood. We shared some similar horror stories and really enjoyed one another's company. I was happy he asked me to share his season ticket. He seemed pleased to meet a female who appeared to understand AND ENJOY THE SPORT of American football.

My date knew about my MS, but he did not totally understand the ramifications of the disease. It was too early in our relationship to open a discussion full of something I didn't understand totally myself.

Talk about a surefire way to scare a guy away!

"Hi, my name is Lisa. I like football and enjoy drinking beer. Oh, by the way I have an incurable neurological disease that will probably sabotage any type of intimate relationship we could ever possibly have, so do not get too close or expect this to continue on as a normal relationship because I have no idea what the future holds for me. Let's go, Mountaineers!"

It was all good, though. It was a beautiful day. I was going to see my favorite college football team. And I was on the arm of a gorgeous fellow. Life is good.

Oh, and it was incredibly hot outside.

My date was aware of my aversion to heat, but I had assured him I would hydrate myself and seek shade as much as possible. Surely, I could walk the half mile from our tailgate parking to our seats in the stadium.

That's me. No Fear.

And I almost made it.

Standing in line for my turn to enter the main gate, a familiar tingling started snaking itself up my right arm. I transferred my game ticket to my left hand when my right hand went numb. The promise of a cooler, and shaded, environment was right beyond that gate. I could see it. I could smell the kettle corn. I could hear the crowd.

But I couldn't feel my ticket float to the ground as I fell (rather unattractively) against my very attractive date.

Next thing I know, I am leaning against a refreshingly cool concrete wall while a young university student wipes my brow with a wet cloth. My date had gone to retrieve a cool drink for me and this angel in the colors of my alma matre waited with me. God bless you, angel.

Wow. Do not dare to criticize the youth of today. They are good. They are angels.

When my date returned with a jumbo, icy lemonade, I was beginning to recover. He suggested we go home. He didn't mind. (But, I could see in his eyes that he really, kinda did.) I suggested he go on to our seats and I would follow when all my limbs had regained their strength. He suggested I must be nuts. He wasn't leaving me.

I fell in love.

We actually saw kick off from our nose-bleed seats and I cooled off enough to enjoy the game. And my date. And the rest of the day.

Heat sucks. It gets me every time.

As documented in the previous chapter, we all fight our personal kryptonite. And sometimes these nasties interchange.

When I am not battling Heat/Humidity, I keep a close eye on Stress. He's a sneaky one. Stress often bides his time in attacking us. Just when we are wiping our brow with success, Stress slaps the back of our head with a delayed counter attack.

At least that's been my experience. Suddenly I find myself in a puddle of gooey MS symptoms when there should be no reason for that. Stress reinforces its arsenal while we celebrate what we think is a job well done.

Here is where I really, really wish I had a mouthy parrot to warn me.

Oh, well.

Oh, by the way. About that gorgeous football date? He is now my husband. He and my son and I live happily ever after in a gold and blue themed stone cottage fully equipped with central air conditioning. Life is good.

Chapter Eleven

Blue, blue, my world is blue...

I fell in love with the OPI nail color Russian Navy after reading the true story of a West Virginia mid-wife who wore this particular hue on her toe-nails, hidden beneath her hospital shoes. It was her own little indulgent secret. As a serious-minded medical professional, she knew the importance of owning a part of herself that was not privy to her public. Her Russian Navy pedicure reminded her that she was still her own person, even when the demands of her professional life dictated responsibilities above and beyond what defined her outside of the office.

Until the turn of the century, nail color was typically feminine in hue: roses, reds, corals. The fashion world took a turn of its own with the birth of the new millennium. Women of all stature and social status embraced the allure of futuristic design. I felt it abnormal to sport powder blues and grassy green on my finger nails and I was certain this was a fashion mistake that would run its course and disappear as quickly as it had come. My grandmother would have an absolute fit if she knew I turned my back on Estee Lauder and agreed to display this crayon-style grooming.

But, I got curious. As long as I kept my feet covered, no one was the wiser of my little secret. It took some getting used to, but my blue pedicure was kind of fun and I only exposed it to public criticism during the summer months, until my position as a public school teacher resumed in the fall. Then, my manicure remained a professional French white tip or a subtle pink.

I remember when I graduated from college with my education degree, there were certain expectations to live by. We were not allowed to wear large or hoop earrings. Our skirts were expected to rest at, or below, knee length. No one dyed their hair in drastic or extreme styles. Visible tattoos were forbidden.

Well, I still wear the appropriate skirt length, maintain a rather boring hair style and I do not possess any tattoos, visible or not. I try to look professional in respect to my college degree. I am a teacher and I need to exhibit the pride that accompanies my position.

After thirty plus years of teaching, I remain steadfast in my beliefs, but I also realize the best way to reach the age group with which I deal is to represent someone with whom they can relate. Even with Russian Navy nails, I am still the teacher and the one in control, but I can still have a little fun with fashion.

The first time my dad saw my dark blue toe nails, he thought they were bruised, that my son had run over my feet with his four-wheeler. I didn't tell him at the time I kind of liked the comparison of being bruised. I have felt bruised for thirteen years. Between the beating of my personal pride and the war my body has taken against my mind, MS has attacked every single inch of my person. It leaves its ugly, if not always visible, bruises daily. That is the figurative bruising, but when I began injecting Beta Seron, the physical bruising became apparent.

Each injection, no matter how careful I execute the procedure, always left a telling mark that often was mistaken as a badge of physical abuse. Top that with the actual abuse my body received at my own hand. The falls, the stumbling, the collisions…all because my feet and my legs refused to follow my lead. Yes, MS bruises me every day.

My Russian Navy nails are a reminder I have a choice in the way I live with MS. It is my self-inflicted bruise and it reminds me to meet each bruise and bump with my chosen reaction to the situation. And hopefully, my new fashion choice will provide an easier conversation topic. One that steers away from all of those unplanned bruises that often receive suspicious stares and hurtful comments.

Maybe it is a character flaw, but my family is full of pride and that sense of pride has been instilled in me and my brothers to the point we do not talk about our personal failings or physical ailment. The less others know about me, the less there is to talk about in small town gossip circuits. Out of sight, out of mind. That's my motto. Maybe my nails are a weird hue, but if that is what holds those wagging tongues attention, it is certainly better than being the target of whispering speculation.

Every day is a new adventure in the war against the MonSter. In the words of Forrest Gump, "Life is like a box of chocolates. You never know what you're going to get."

MS holds that same mystery. One day I might energetically walk miles with my BFF, the good ol Wii, after which my cat and I might perform twenty minutes of body and soul stretching Yoga. It will feel good.

Unfortunately, the despised chocolate covered cherry (I hate them) lurks around the corner of every forward step we take. An hour after all of this wonderful endorphin-fueled activity, the vision might blur or the hand tremors begin.

MS takes planning. We must plan for the unexpected.

On a relapse morning it is necessary to shelve the most recent good feelings in favor of a less strenuous day.

I never thought I might one day play host to a life-altering disease, so I really did not know how to react to the news I had one. I am still shocked every time I am reminded of my affliction.

Multiple Sclerosis is an unpredictable disease that affects its targets in different ways. MS is not partial to age, race, or gender. It offers no favors to the young or weak at heart.

I do not have many complaints since my diagnosis. I have met several comrades in this disease and I thank God daily for blessing me with the ability to tolerate my physical existence in a relatively unchanged manner. I do tire more easily, but, hey, that's part of growing older. Common Sense is by my side to remind me to keep things in perspective.

Never would I make light of this increasingly publicized disease, but I live with MS and I choose to do so in a positive manner. Sitting around moaning about it will not change the reality of what it is. I admit I am not as pro-active as I probably should be, but I do stay aware of medical research. I believe in staying informed, but I have never felt it necessary to bombard myself with medical reports and the politics of owning a disease.

There is no reason NOT to indulge myself in little gifts of humanity along the way. When finances allow it, I get a mani/pedi every now and then to remind myself that I am worthy, I am beautiful, I am a member of the human race. (Besides, Super Heroes need to maintain their outward appearance, right?)

So, treat yourself to that Russian Navy manicure. Make a hair appointment. Indulge in a Starbucks Mocha Latte. Spend an hour (or more) with a good book.

The Monster, unfortunately, is here to stay. That doesn't mean we must give it ALL of our attention ALL of the time.

Chapter Twelve

Not tonight, dear, I have a headache.

This lovely July morning dawned in a typical fashion of early fall design. The air was crisp and I could smell the distinction of football in the air. Kind of weird for July, but West Virginia is not known for playing by the weather rules of nature.

Regardless, it was the perfect morning for chores. I cleaned out my closet in record time, put dinner in the crock pot for later, and even enjoyed twenty minutes of gentle yoga, all before my teenage son even bothered to address the day from his dark bedroom.

I felt great.

And, then the bomb dropped.

As I was preparing to take a shower, my head began to thump dully and my vision blurred around the edges. Before I could decide on the color of my wash cloth, I knew I had a migraine, full blown and very, very unexpected.

I have always been prone to headaches, but since my diagnosis and maybe because of it, when I experience a headache it absolutely ruins an otherwise wonderful day.

And these were no normal headaches. It is an extreme hangover sensation from days left on college campus. There is no way to explain the pain, the nausea, the dizziness that accompanies these headaches. And there is no way to outlast them. Drugs are necessary and immediate.

Thank goodness I have the luxury of my teacher's summer holiday, as well, the ability to down my extra strength ibuprofen and recline on the couch to close my eyes and try to relax. A cool cloth over the eyes and I am set.

I hate headaches, especially these of the "hangover" variety and especially when I didn't even get to imbibe something yummy the night before that would result in such pain. I was never into the marijuana that many of my friends experimented with when we were younger and some still do to this day. It is a way of life for some people and I know several folks who would love to move to Colorado if they could.

Pot never turned me on and use of anything like that has always scared me. So, in my research of MS, I have yet to understand the effects smoking pot has on multiple sclerosis. Evidently marijuana offers respite from MS pain. I refuse to judge anyone who uses pot for medical reasons. We all must discover our own weapon to battle our kryptonite. We do what we need to do and there is no disgrace in that. It is just not my thing.

But at that moment, I would have "passed the pipe" to extinguish the pain in my head.

Probably more than the intense pain, I hated the suddenness and unexpectedness of the arrival of my pain. There was no indication that it was coming. It just arrived like an unwelcome guest and there was no polite way to let it know it was not welcome. And even with the attitude of complete indifference to its presence, it refused to take the hint. It was oblivious of my disdain for its existence and it totally ignored my attempts to kick it out the door. Aren't ignorant guests fun?

So, as I reclined on my couch, full of prescription pain killers, cool cloth on my eyes and my twitchy feet elevated on cushions….yes, now my lower extremities were involved. Somehow my brain got the message out and everyone was invited to this little pain fest.

My drop foot, even though elevated and not on the floor, refused to remain on the sofa and kept flopping over the side and onto the floor. I mean, really. Had all of my muscles gone on strike? Why could something as simple and elementary as keeping one's legs stretched out before them become such a chore? But that is what MS is all about.

Then I realized what was happening. MS had been stalking me and teasing me all morning by allowing my body to return to things gone past. I had walked across the room with no stumbling. My mind was clear and I was full of energy prior to the arrival of head pain. I had been duped and MS was ready to crown itself victorious. I couldn't help but to raise my invisible glass to this worthy opponent to allow it to wallow in its success for a few more seconds.

Game well played, my friend. I could feel the effects of 800 milligrams of ibuprofen coming to my rescue. In rebellion of my screaming head, I reached for the television remote and fired up the infomercial on channel whatever. I mentally apologized to still sleeping teenage son, but shook my mental fist at MS.

Take that, head pain, because I can. And I will.

And now to the nitty gritty, X-rated stuff...

I don't know how guys with MS handle this, but there are times when I must avoid intimate contact with my husband at all cost. And it has nothing to do with lack of desire. It has everything to do with FEAR.

What if I pee on him? Or worse? (Because "that" happens also. Yuck!)

Incontinence has played a huge role in my MS identity. Remember the traffic light? Incontinence is difficult to talk about, not to mention a real sexual turn-off.

Add to the possibility of a bed-wetting session, there is the existence of the woman parts going completely numb. Yep. That's fun. And when he hears me writhing in discomfort, he only hears lustful bliss.

I never want my husband to feel rejected, but I also need to maintain my own dignity.

Wow, isn't having MS enough of a challenge without the need to comfort our loved ones?

Worry = Stress = Disaster

And I have worried and stressed enough about this issue of intimacy. So, work it out on your own.

Communicate with your partner. Own your kryptonite, but don't let it own you. You may borrow my Common Sense if you want.

Because that's all I have to say about that.

Chapter Thirteen

I'd like to buy a P.

I've learned my MS has made me rather obsessive. I obsess about my son's future, what to prepare for evening meal, going to the grocery store, keeping a clean house, retirement…all in a day's agenda. Add the bonus of the silent, hidden issues credited to MS. With this added pressure, my obsessions take on a much more cynical attitude.

Because my drop foot forces me to assume an exaggerated gait, I am constantly looking for obstacles in my path. Anything can interrupt my walking, from the tiniest pebble to the most obvious barrier. Drop foot restrains me from putting on my trousers one leg at a time. I cannot force my right foot to lift itself up to meet the trouser leg opening.

Oops. I'm preaching to the choir, aren't I?

Therefore, I have become rather obsessive about caring for my drop foot and that means exercise, exercise, exercise. I have learned that it is not all about just the foot. Drop foot needs to be looked at all the way up to the hip. Those are the muscles that actually control the movement of the foot.

Not everyone reacts as favorably to steroid treatment as I do, so as with medicinal marijuana, this may not be for you. MS friends have relayed periods of severe moodiness, depression and even destructive anger while taking steroids. I know one lady who would rather exist in physical pain than undergo the emotional swing that steroids play on her.

I, on the other hand, am euphoric when prescribed Prednisone. I can walk. I am sure-footed and not afraid of steps without aid and I even walk briskly. My balance is spot on and my energy level excels. And my mood! Wow! I am transported to my carefree, fun-loving 20s pre-MS. I am invincible when taking prednisone. I can truly understand the allure of DRUG addiction and I do NOT understand why I cannot feel this way all of the time. It is not fair.

What is in Prednisone that cannot be packaged as THE MS drug?

Every time I wean myself from a cycle of Prednisone, I liken myself to the main character in a story I read long ago.

In *Flowers for Algernon* by Daniel Keyes, Charlie Gordon is a middle-aged man with an IQ of 60. Due to his exceptional work ethic, sincere desire to learn and the fact he has no living relatives, Charlie is accepted into an experimental program to alter his learning capabilities.

Charlie has an "opurashun," followed by exhausting strategies to increase his intelligence. He maintains a journal to record his progress and opinions of his development. Charlie triples his IQ but learns his exceptional gift is as much a handicap as the inability to clearly connect with the world around him. Upon the conclusion of the experiment, his intellectual progress reverses and he finds himself at a lower IQ than before. Not entirely understanding this reversal of fortune, Charlie grieves for the unfamiliar abilities the surgery and experiment allowed him.

That's how I deal every time I am presented with a Prednisone experience. I realize my super human powers (all of which are just considered normal for most people) are to be short-lived and I will pay a price at the end of treatment.

But it's good while it lasts.

Gee, I just kinda made myself sad.

Chapter Fourteen

Bruised, But Not Broken

Sometimes I wake in the middle of the night, thinking about my MS and how it affects my life and the lives of those around me. I really believe the effects of this disease began long before I was aware of its existence: the tingling in my fingers and arms when I learned to play raquet ball in college; the times when I fell over my own feet for no reason…even long ago and far away in my teen years; the experiences with memory loss that were in no way related to late-night beer bashes. These were all red flags begging for attention. I just had no idea what kind of attention to offer.

Super Heroes get banged around a lot, but on the big screen their scrapes and bruises heal and fade quickly. The scars the MonSter inflicts on us are not so easily corrected. We do not possess the cinematic or comic book illustrator to "fix" us.

During my latest research I found that an estimated 1 in 3 children are diagnosed with MS symptoms. Does that mean I might have been carting around this inconvenient condition for much longer than I could guess?

I really do believe my hand numbness and aversion to heat might have been early MS indicators, but that doesn't explain all those years of sun worshipping I enjoyed while life guarding in my youth. I do not recall any episode of numbness or dizziness occurring in all of those years. Does that mean those years of severe heat exposure could have possibly been an accelerant to the diagnosis of the disease? Did my child hood illnesses of measles, mumps, and chicken pox contribute to my diagnosis? What about the unexpected bout of hepatitis I contracted in the fourth grade after sharing a licorice stick with an infected classmate? Does one disease lead to another?

And there are the zillion questions concerning MS progression that attacks different individuals. Why did a former art teacher, a retired doctor, and a friend's mother all die as a result of the disease? Especially when it is well publicized that one CANNOT DIE from MS? Why am I ambling along with a stumbling gait when the mother of young children is in a wheelchair?

I just do NOT understand this disease. There is no rhyme nor reason for it.

Did you know that years ago individuals experiencing what we currently recognize as MS symptoms were actually institutionalized or even punished as being in cohorts with the devil? (I know I keep mentioning this. I am absolutely fascinated with this detail, as well as in awe of the progression of medical science.)

Well, if there was ever a devilish disease, this is it. I definitely do not want to be tried as a witch, though! At least not for exhibiting traits of multiple sclerosis!

Multiple Sclerosis robs us of precious moments in our day-to-day lives. My dear friend, Jamie (love ya like a sis!) was robbed of many joys as a direct result of her lack of mobility. Additional health issues, as a result of the existence of MS, stole her away from her son and loving husband. She will not physically participate in the many milestones that make any parent proud and most children happy for a loving mother.

My own son often verbalizes his concern that I am doing okay. He has gone out of his way to help me carry things to and from the car. He has reminded me to take a few minutes to rest while he has also urged me to spend some time exercising (He, of the great dark cave of his computer lab bedroom.) He doesn't say it, but I can see the FEAR in his eyes.

My love for him is so great that I just shudder when I imagine not being "there" for him. If I was forced to sit at home while he receives an honor, play in the championship game, or pose for prom pictures,

I would be crushed. I can only imagine the disappointments my friend suffered.

Yes, MS stinks; but we do not have to bow down to its ugliness. Just sayin.'

When I think of my dear sweet friend, I am truly overwhelmed with the definition of unfair and how unkind multiple sclerosis can be. Jamie was several years younger than I, a former gymnast and an incredibly beautiful girl. Shortly after diagnosis, her mobility went under attack, forcing her physical health to suffer. She could no longer walk, control a steady hand with which to feed herself, or care for her family.

I miss her every day.

But not as much as her husband and children miss her.

Multiple Sclerosis is a thief. It poetically comes at night and sucks the marrow from its victims. That is why we must be Super Heroes. We will fight 'til the end. And we will make it all count.

I recently read the following statement in a MS publication:

"I was diagnosed with multiple sclerosis in the spring of 2005 and have since learned many lessons about living well with a chronic illness. The most important lesson I have learned, however, is to be your own advocate. No one knows you better than you. In order to be the best possible advocate for yourself, you need to educate yourself on your disease, as well as the ins and outs of the healthcare system. Research doctors and therapists who can help you, communicate openly and effectively with your healthcare providers, and most importantly – never give up hope. You are worth fighting for!"

Well said. Tis a shame these words are so true. We are our own advocates because when it comes right down to the nitty gritty, no one really knows the limits of our body more than we know ourselves. I appreciate the individuals who have studied medical science and concentrated on neurological medicine, but they can only speculate if they are not experiencing the same life altering symptoms their patients are.

When I was initially diagnosed, my attending neurologist was in the process of training a current intern and, with my consent, this marvelous young man and I formed a bond I will always equate with the positive attitude I developed early on. He held my hand (literally and figuratively) when he performed my first ever spinal tap and he made me comfortable with my diagnosis. He didn't have all the answers, but his youthful enthusiasm secured in me the promise that he would go to the ends of the earth to bring me any information he could obtain.

Maybe it was because this was all so new and so very, very scary to me, but I fell in love with this man and his encouragement. Not in a romantic sense, no. But I just knew that if there was anyone on the planet who was going to take care of me, soon-to-be Dr. Lewis was the man.

Not everyone is fortunate enough to find the support of a caring neurologist. Keep searching, though. He/She is out there. We all need the comfort of an authority figure. The Charlie to our angels, the Batman to our Robin.

We all suffer scars. That's just reality. And we all need a sidekick to lean on. Mine is Common Sense. When in doubt, I rely upon him. God gave us the ability to think things through and it would be the ultimate sin not to take advantage of this gift.

So, yeah, I am bruised and am still bruising. But, I'm not broken.

The Final Chapter...Or, is it?

Multiple Sclerosis is a neurological condition that affects an alarming number of people every day, attacking myelin, which is the protective sheaf that covers the body's nerve endings.

Fortunately, the advancements in medical research have made it possible to treat Multiple Sclerosis rather than turn a deaf ear and a blind eye on those experiencing what was once not recognized as a treatable disease. The reality of this disease has reached international attention with celebrity announcements by Montel Williams and Ann Romney.

Currently, the National Multiple Sclerosis Society sponsors fundraising awareness campaigns in the form of organized walks, running events, and cycling marathons. As a member of the National Multiple Sclerosis Society, members receive free and informative literature as well as the latest news on advancements in a Cure. (No, I am not an undercover agent for the society and, no, they are not paying me to provide free advertisement. I just truly believe in their dedication to learning more about the MonSter.)

Researchers and clinicians dedicated to the study of Multiple Sclerosis have categorized MS into four disease routes.

I have Relapsing-remitting MS (RRMS), which is the initial diagnosis for approximately 85% of persons identified with MS. This is where it all begins and I pray daily this is where it ends for me. I do not want my MS to progress any further. It is bad enough where it is.

Secondary-progressive MS (SPMS) occurs in roughly 50% of those individuals initially diagnosed with PRMS and is identified approximately 10-25 years after initial diagnosis.

Primary-Progressive MS (PPMS) basically progresses very quickly without any relapse or remission. Roughly 10% of persons diagnosed with MS suffer from PPMS. My dear, dear Jamie battled PPMS. PPMS is a formidable foe that literally blind-sided Jamie. In one moment she was diagnosed with a condition that we compared often and just as quickly we had very little to compare in the way of similarities. I often felt guilty because my MS was so much more benign than hers. It sometimes felt like we were suffering from two totally different conditions. And, I guess in a way, we were.

Progressive-relapsing MS (PRMS) affects approximately 5% of folks diagnosed with MS. Although PRMS is a progressive form of the MonSter, its victims may experience intermittent relapses.

The authors of *Multiple Sclerosis for Dummies* refer to Multiple Sclerosis as a personal "thumbprint." MS is an extremely personalized disease with an expansive variety of attack plans. As Warriors on our Super Hero path, we are different, yet there is no kryptonite that separates us in battle against the MonSter.

I do not have all the answers. I do not even know a tenth of the answers, but that doesn't stop me from learning daily. My treatment plan fluctuates often. But that is what research is all about, right? Currently I am toying with essential oils and they are awesome. Next month I might look into acupuncture. Massage is expensive but so worth breaking into the piggy bank for. I will not tell you to do the same. I can only suggest and share my own experience.

My hope is that this humble offering might touch a fellow MSer and inspire my comrades in our MS Super Hero family to continue moving forward.

This may be the final chapter in this publication, but this NOT the final chapter in my life.

To be continued…

Stay strong, don't be sorry, that's what we MS WARRIORS ARE HERE FOR! So vent on, ears and the heart will remain open! But suicide is not an **Option for any of us. That's giving up and not trusting in God. That will never be me! What about you all? Maybe you have to change your meds, comminicate all with your doctor, with your MS family is good because we're great, but we're not the professionals!** #REALWARRIORSSTAYFOCUSSED and #THEWEAKWARRIORSWORKHARDERONBECOMINGSTRONG

—Michelle Staton West

My Go-To's:

Multiple Sclerosis for Dummies by Rosalind Kalb, PH. D., Barbara Giesser, MD, and Kathleen Costello, ANP-BC.

MYMSYOGA with Baron Baptiste and Dr. Eliot Frohman can be found on www.MyMSYoga.com or call 1-800-456-2255.

Yoga Zone: Gentle Yoga for Beginners was published in 2003 by Koch Vision. I do not know where I found this, but it is a very user friendly DVD. www.kochvision.com

If you have a Wii, the Wii Fit Plus program is an awesome way to exercise and record your progress. The avatars on the program even celebrate with you and encourage you along the way!

We're Not Drunk. We Have MS! Facebook page. Battle on, Warriors!

Please, please contact me if you want to talk more.
LisaAnnetteMcCombs@yahoo.com
I am also on Facebook.
Or you can do it the old-fashioned way:
Lisa A. McCombs
358 McCue Avenue
Monongah, WV 26554